Handbook of Treatment Planning in Radiation Oncology

GW00503340

Handbook of Treatment Planning in Radiation Oncology

Second Edition

Editors

Gregory M. M. Videtic, MD, CM, FRCPC
Staff Physician
Department of Radiation Oncology
Taussig Cancer Institute
Cleveland Clinic;
Associate Professor of Medicine
Cleveland Clinic Lerner College of Medicine of Case Western
    Reserve University
Cleveland, Ohio

Neil M. Woody, MD
Resident Physician
Department of Radiation Oncology
Taussig Cancer Institute
Cleveland Clinic
Cleveland, Ohio

Associate Editor
Andrew D. Vassil, MD
Associate Staff Physician
Department of Radiation Oncology
Taussig Cancer Institute
Cleveland Clinic;
Clinical Assistant Professor of Medicine
Cleveland Clinic Lerner College of Medicine of Case Western Reserve University
Cleveland, Ohio

demosMEDICAL

New York

Visit our website at www.demosmedical.com

ISBN: 9781620700358
e-book ISBN: 9781617051975

Acquisitions Editor: Rich Winters
Compositor: S4Carlisle Publishing Services

Medicine is an ever-changing science. Research and clinical experience are continually expanding our knowledge, in particular our understanding of proper treatment and drug therapy. The authors, editors, and publisher have made every effort to ensure that all information in this book is in accordance with the state of knowledge at the time of production of the book. Nevertheless, the authors, editors, and publisher are not responsible for errors or omissions or for any consequences from application of the information in this book and make no warranty, expressed or implied, with respect to the contents of the publication. Every reader should examine carefully the package inserts accompanying each drug and should carefully check whether the dosage schedules mentioned therein or the contraindications stated by the manufacturer differ from the statements made in this book. Such examination is particularly important with drugs that are either rarely used or have been newly released on the market.

Library of Congress Cataloging-in-Publication Data

Handbook of treatment planning in radiation oncology / editors, Gregory M.M. Videtic, Neil Woody ; associate editor, Andrew D. Vassil. -- Second edition.
    p. ; cm.
  Includes bibliographical references and index.
  ISBN 978-1-62070-035-8 — ISBN 1-62070-035-2 — ISBN 978-1-61705-197-5 (e-book)
  I. Videtic, Gregory M. M., editor. II. Woody, Neil, editor.
  [DNLM: 1. Neoplasms—radiotherapy--Handbooks. 2. Patient Care Planning—Handbooks.
3. Planning Techniques—Handbooks. QZ 39]
  RC271.R3
  616.99'40642--dc23
                                                                    2014010745

Printed in the United States of America by Bang Printing.
14 15 16 17 / 5 4 3 2 1

Contents

Preface to the Second Edition

As I write this preface to the second edition, I can easily recall that our only focus when working on the original *Handbook of Treatment Planning in Radiation Oncology* was getting it done right and on schedule! Now we find ourselves on the threshold of completing a revised and updated version of this manual, and that fact truly exceeds any of our initial expectations. Indeed, the response to the first handbook has been humbling. Whether it was the numerous testimonials on how helpful it was (from both trainees and seasoned professionals), its translation into other languages, or it being listed as "sold out" at a professional meeting: All provided strong validation of the utility and quality of our work. Grateful for those accolades, we approached the present project no differently than the last, with a strong sense of responsibility and discipline.

The second edition of the handbook maintains the principles of the first. To begin with, this remains a focused pocket-sized reference to act as a quick resource to those engaged in the steps of radiation therapy planning and delivery. Second, it continues to be descriptive in outlook and not prescriptive, given the ongoing evolution in radiation oncology practice. Lastly, it aims to complement, but not replace, the judgment of the competent professional who is involved in an individual patient's care. All chapters were carefully reviewed and, where indicated, content was corrected or updated.

New topics are formally introduced when it is clear that an understanding of their planning process is becoming part of routine practice, as, for example, with the use of stereotactic body radiotherapy in the treatment of liver malignancies. In other situations, mention without extensive detail was felt appropriate, as the modality remains investigational or under limited use: An example would be proton therapy for lung cancer.

This edition of the *Handbook of Treatment Planning in Radiation Oncology* continues the tradition of excellence from our residents and effective mentorship of our trainees by staff that is a hallmark of our department. Now, a new generation of residents, working with new and previous staff physician authors, exemplifies this commitment. Dr. Andrew Vassil, my previous coeditor, kindly provided encouragement and support throughout this project, despite his responsibilities as a clinician and director of one of our satellite practices. His earlier editorial role was now ably and enthusiastically filled by Dr. Neil Woody, a junior resident, whose leadership skills, hard work, and diligence ensured completion of this exciting project.

Gregory M. M. Videtic, MD, CM, FRCPC

Preface to the First Edition

The past decade has seen rapid changes in the field of radiation oncology, ranging from an increasing shift to "evidence-based" treatments, to a constantly expanding technological armamentarium. In this setting, the discipline's reference literature has also blossomed, with a large variety of clinically-oriented textbooks and manuals becoming available to meet the needs both of busy trainees and clinicians engaged in the care of patients with cancer. For all that, radiation oncology remains a "technical" discipline, whose practice is gradually learned through experience, as it is handed down from "master to apprentice," typically in the familiar setting of the simulator room. Mindful of this, discussions with our residents at the Cleveland Clinic had suggested that there was a need for a focused pocket-sized handbook to act as quick resource for them as they carried out the steps during the planning and delivery of radiation therapy.

Handbook of Treatment Planning in Radiation Oncology is intended to be descriptive and not prescriptive. No treatment or equipment recommendations are being endorsed. Clinical stage descriptions employed the TNM definitions of the sixth edition of the *AJCC Cancer Staging Handbook*. In setting down the steps to follow in the treatment planning of an individual patient, there is no intent at providing comprehensive clinical algorithms for treatment decision-making. Rather, we have assumed that the indications for a particular therapy are known, and therefore, our focus is on a series of suggested steps to follow to successfully complete effective radiotherapy planning. Sections are organized by body site or system, whichever proved best for consistency in presenting the general principles of planning; for example, the chapter on thoracic malignancies includes esophageal cancers. We have also presented specialized topics such as palliative therapy and pediatrics. After referencing general planning requirements, each specific subsite within a given section then provides more specific details on approaches to radiotherapy planning. Although drawn from the wealth of clinical experience at our institution and the copious notes of the residents, numerous sources were referenced and reviewed to present the most up-to-date standards in our discipline. Recognizing that almost every component of radiation treatment can be considered an active area of investigation, we have deliberately limited our planning recommendations to what would be considered good and safe practice at this point. The detailed protocols available online from the Radiation Therapy Oncology Group (RTOG) were invaluable in providing structure and a model for outlining the steps in good radiotherapy planning. Ultimately, the practice of radiation oncology is an art—nothing can replace experience and many clinicians may debate the finer points in any given section. That said, guidelines provide structure and like a phrase book for a foreign language, they help put (sometimes) unknown or disparate terms together to form an intelligible concept. The competent professional will know when to move beyond these recommendations as required for individual patient care.

Handbook of Treatment Planning in Radiation Oncology represents the diligent efforts of our residents working under the guidance and mentorship of staff physicians. The quality of their chapters, their collaborative spirit, and their prompt response to feedback made the experience of editing their submissions a pleasure. The technical contributions of Nicole Pavelecky, CMD, staff dosimetrist, were invaluable in producing consistent images of high quality. Last but certainly not least, this project would not have been realized without the tireless dedication and outstanding contributions of Dr. Andrew Vassil, senior resident, and my coeditor.

Gregory M. M. Videtic, MD, CM, FRCPC
Andrew D. Vassil, MD

Contributors

All contributors of this text are affiliated with the Department of Radiation Oncology, Cleveland Clinic, Cleveland, Ohio.

May Abdel-Wahab, MD

Samuel T. Chao, MD

Sheen Cherian, MD

John F. Greskovich, Jr, MD

Jason W. D. Hearn, MD

Edward W. Jung, MD

Jeffrey A. Kittel, MD

Rupesh R. Kotecha, MD

Shlomo A. Koyfman, MD

Aryavarta M. S. Kumar, MD, PhD

Roger M. Macklis, MD

Anthony L. Magnelli, MS

Gaurav Marwaha, MD

Erin S. Murphy, MD

Steven C. Oh, MD

Nicole Pavelecky, CMD

Monica E. Shukla, MD

Kevin L. Stephans, MD

Abigail L. Stockham, MD

John H. Suh, MD

Rahul D. Tendulkar, MD

Andrew D. Vassil, MD

Gregory M. M. Videtic, MD, CM, FRCPC

Michael A. Weller, MD

Neil M. Woody, MD

Handbook of Treatment Planning in Radiation Oncology

1 General Physics Principles

Andrew D. Vassil, Nicole Pavelecky,
Anthony L. Magnelli, and Gregory M. M. Videtic

GENERAL PRINCIPLES

- Percent depth dose (PDD) is the ratio of absorbed dose (on the central axis) at a chosen depth to the absorbed dose at the reference depth D_{max}.
- Normalizing dose refers to setting a desired dose point to which all other dose points are referred. For example, if one chooses to normalize to the D_{max} point, then all other points within the patient will receive a lesser dose (ie, the 100% isodose line is set to D_{max}).
- Isodose lines are lines of equal dose overlaid on a patient's planning images. Isodose lines can be displayed in absolute dose, or normalized to a reference point (eg, the calculation point or isocenter).
- Depth dose (DD) is a function of
  - Energy: as energy increases, DD increases
  - Depth: as depth increases, DD decreases
  - Source-surface distance (SSD): as SSD increases, DD decreases
  - Field size: as field size increases, DD increases (due to increased scatter)
- D_{max} increases (moves deeper in the patient) as field size decreases. This is due to an increase in effective energy, as there is less collimator scatter, patient scatter, and transmission through the thicker portion of the flattening filter.

- "Hot spots"
  - Classically defined as a high-dose region of up to +10% in the treatment volume
  - Tend to increase in size as separation increases (eg, comparing plans on patients with a small versus large body mass index)
- Isodose lines shift as tissue electron density changes. This is accounted for by "heterogeneity correction," for example, isodose lines move away from the surface when beam goes through air and are brought toward the surface when beam goes through bone.
- Source-surface distance (SSD) represents the distance between the radiation source and the treatment surface.
- Source-axis distance (SAD) represents the distance between the radiation source and the axis (isocenter) about which the table, gantry, and collimator rotate.

TARGET VOLUMES

International Commission on Radiation Units & Measurements (ICRU) 50: "Prescribing, Recording, and Reporting Photon Beam Therapy"

- Gross tumor volume (GTV): gross palpable or visible/demonstrable extent and location of malignant growth.
- Clinical target volume (CTV): Volume that contains the GTV and/or a subclinical microscopic malignant disease that has to be eliminated.
- Planning target volume (PTV): geometrical concept. Defined to select appropriate beam sizes and beam arrangements, taking into consideration the net effect of all the possible geometrical variations and inaccuracies to ensure that the prescribed dose is actually absorbed in the CTV. Its size and shape not only depend on the CTV but also on the treatment technique used to compensate for the effects of organ and patient movement and inaccuracies in beam and patient setup.
- Treated volume: volume enclosed by an isodose surface (eg, 95% isodose), selected and specified as being appropriate in achieving the purpose of treatment. Ideally, treated volume would be identical to PTV but may also be considerably larger than PTV.
- Irradiated volume: tissue volume that receives a dose that is considered significant in relation to normal tissue tolerance. Dose should be expressed either in absolute values or relative to the specified dose to the PTV.
- Integral dose: a measure of the total energy absorbed in the treated volume.
- Organs at risk (OAR): normal tissues with radiation sensitivity that may significantly influence treatment planning and/or prescribed dose.

TREATMENT PLANNING

Plan Evaluation

- Review of the dose-volume histogram (DVH), maximum doses, minimum doses, mean doses, and isodose distribution on all axial images (high- and low-isodose lines) is essential when reviewing plans.
  - *D percentage*: allows the analysis of a dose (*D*) that encompasses a percentage of a volume of interest (eg, D100, D90, and D80 represent the dose encompassing 100%, 90%, and 80% of a volume of interest, respectively).
  - *V percentage*: allows the analysis of a percent volume (*V*) that receives a particular dose (eg, V100, V90, and V80 represent the percent of a volume of interest that receives 100%, 90%, and 80% of the prescribed dose, respectively).

ICRU 50: "Prescribing, Recording, and Reporting Photon Beam Therapy" Recommendations for Reporting Dose

- ICRU reference point
  - Dose at the point should be clinically relevant and representative of the dose throughout PTV.
  - The point should be easy to define in a clear and unambiguous way.
  - The point should be selected where the dose can be accurately determined (physical accuracy).
  - The point should be selected in a region where there is no steep dose gradient.
  - The point should be located at the center of the PTV and, when possible, at the intersection of the beam axes.
  - The dose at the ICRU reference point is the ICRU reference dose.
- Dose at/near center of PTV, maximum dose to PTV, and minimum dose to PTV should always be reported.
- Maximum dose: highest dose in PTV. A volume is considered clinically meaningful if its minimum diameter exceeds 15 mm; however, if it occurs in a small organ (eg, the eye, optic nerve, larynx), a dimension smaller than 15 mm has to be considered.
- Minimum dose: lowest dose in PTV. In contrast to maximum dose, no volume limit is recommended.
- "Hot spots": volume that receives dose larger than 100% of the specified PTV dose. In general, a "hot spot" is considered significant only if the minimum diameter exceeds 15 mm; however, if it occurs in a small organ (eg, the eye, optic nerve, larynx), a dimension smaller than 15 mm has to be considered.

ICRU 62 "Prescribing, Recording, and Reporting Photon Beam Therapy (Supplement to ICRU Report 50)"

Global concept and definition of PTV is not changed, but the definition is supplemented.

- Internal margin (IM): variations in size, shape, and position of the CTV relative to anatomic reference points (eg, filling of bladder, movements of respiration). The internal variations are physiological ones and result in change in site, size, and shape of the CTV.
- Internal target volume (ITV): volume encompassing the CTV and IM (ITV = CTV + IM).
- Setup margin (SM): uncertainties in patient positioning and alignment of therapeutic beams during treatment planning and through all treatment sessions. The uncertainties may vary with selection of beam geometries and may depend on variations in patient positioning, mechanical uncertainties of the equipment (eg, sagging of gantry, collimators, or couch), dosimetric uncertainties, transfer setup errors from simulator to treatment unit, and human factors. These may vary from center to center and from machine to machine.
- PTV = CTV + IM + SM. The penumbra of the beam(s) is not considered when delineating the PTV. However, when selecting beam sizes, the width of the penumbra has to be taken into account and the beam size adjusted accordingly.
- A dose variation within the treatment volume of between +/−7% is generally accepted.
- Conformity index: treated volume/PTV. It is implied that treated volume completely encompasses the PTV.
- OAR volumes:
  - Planning organ at risk (OAR) volume (PRV): analogous to PTV for OAR. PRV = OAR + IM + SM.
- Dosing
  - Biologically effective dose (BED) calculations are based on the linear quadratic model of radiation effect.
  - BED equations are used to compare various fractionation schemes for their potential effects on early- and late-responding tissues. Depending on the clinical scenario, BED for late effects drives the choice of dose and fraction.
  - α/β ratio represents the inherent sensitivity to fractionation.
  - An α/β ratio of 3 is typically used for late-responding tissues and 10 for early-responding tissues (and most epithelial tumors).

- BED = $(nd) \times [1 + (d/\{\alpha/\beta\})]$, where n is the number of fractions and d is dose per fraction
  - 78 Gy/2 Gy/fx, 39 fx, 5 fx per week.
    Early effects: $(39 \times 2) \times [1 + (2/10)] = 93.6\,\mathrm{Gy}_{10}$
    Late effects: $(39 \times 2) \times [1 + (2/3)] = 130\,\mathrm{Gy}_3$
  - 70 Gy/2.5 Gy/fx, 28 fx, 5 fx per week.
    Early effects: $(28 \times 2.5) \times [1 + (2.5/10)] = 87.5\,\mathrm{Gy}_{10}$
    Late effects: $(28 \times 2.5) \times [1 + (2.5/3)] = 128\,\mathrm{Gy}_3$
- Percentage of normal bone marrow irradiated using standard radiation ports (Table 1.1)
- Block margins versus dosimetric margins
  - Using "block margins," the secondary collimator [cerrobend block or multileaf collimator (MLC)] expands circumferentially beyond the target by a fixed distance ("block margin") as seen by a beam's eye view.
  - Using "dosimetric margins," dose is prescribed to a chosen circumferential expansion around a defined volume.
- Wedges
  - Wedges are tissue compensators.
  - They are used to alter isodose distribution to a defined angle (Figure 1.1).

TABLE 1.1 Percentage of Normal Bone Marrow Irradiated Using Standard Radiation Ports

Site	Marrow Volume at Risk
Skull (not including mandible)	12%
Upper limb girdle (unilateral, including humeral head, scapulae, clavicle)	4%
Sternum	2%
Ribs (all)	8%
Ribs (hemithorax)	4%
Cervical vertebrae (all)	3%
Thoracic vertebrae (all)	14%
Lumbar vertebrae (all)	11%
Sacrum	14%
Pelvis	26%
Mantle field	25%
Upper para-aortic lymph nodes	45%

Data were derived from Ellis RE, *Physics in Medicine and Biology*, Vol. 5, 1961.

FIGURE 1.1 Isodose distribution in a tissue-equivalent phantom using a 6-MV photon field with a 45° physical wedge (10 × 10 cm field size, 100 SAD, isocenter at D_{max}).

- Physical wedges are placed in the beam path to attenuate the beam.
- Dynamic wedge is the movement of the primary collimator while the beam is on to vary intensity across the field.
- A wedged pair is useful for superficial lesions (Figure 1.2)
  - A pair of coplanar beams is designed with wedging to produce a more homogenous isodose distribution.
  - The "heel" of the wedge is placed inward. Wedge angle = 90 − (hinge angle/2); however, determining the optimal wedge angle may require multiple planning trials.
- Field matching
  - At an electron/photon beam interface, the hot spot is just inside the photon beam (due to bulging out of the electron field isodose distribution; see Figure 1.3).
  - Match junction may be shifted every 8 Gy to 10 Gy by 0.5 to 1 cm to minimize cumulative overlap, also known as "feathering the junction."
  - The light field represents the photon 50% isodose line.
- Blocking
  - Field blocking is accomplished through cerrobend blocks and/or multileaf collimators.

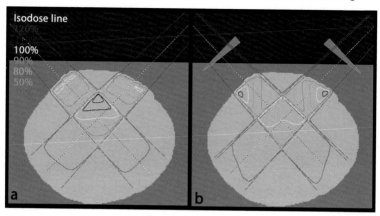

FIGURE 1.2 Isodose distribution in a simulated curved tissue-equivalent phantom using a pair of 6-MV photon fields (10 × 10 cm field size, 100 SAD) (a) showing the influence of 45° physical wedges on isodose distribution (b). The only difference between the figures is the presence of the wedges.

FIGURE 1.3 Example of photon-electron field match in a tissue equivalent phantom. A 6-MV photon field (10 × 10 cm field size, 100 SAD, isocenter at D_{max}) and a 9-MV photon field (10 × 10 cm cone, 100 SAD, isocenter at surface) were normalized to D_{max}.

■ There is approximately 7% to 10% transmission through a half-beam cut block, 4% to 7% through a corner block, and 1% to 2% through the primary collimator (varies due to differences in scatter).
■ Cerrobend is made of bismuth, tin, lead, and cadmium.
■ A half value layer (HVL) is the amount of attenuating material that allows 50% transmission.
■ HVL increases with depth due to "beam hardening" (ie, attenuation of lower energy photons).
■ Intensity remaining (transmission): 10% transmission through 3.3 HVL, 1% through 6.6 HVL, and 0.1% after 10 HVL.

■ Bolus
  ■ Bolus material is used to increase surface dose through beam interaction before a beam enters a patient.
  ■ Its electron density should be similar to that of tissue.
  ■ Synthetic materials are available, and alternatives include paraffin wax, towels soaked in water, and ultrasound gel in a bag.

SELECTED TECHNICAL FACTS

■ Beam characteristics (Table 1.2)
■ Photon and electron beam central axis PDD curves for selected energies (Figure 1.4a and b)
■ Representative isodose distributions for selected posteroanterior (PA) and anteroposterior/posteroanterior (AP/PA) photon fields (Figures 1.5 and 1.6)
■ Isodose distributions of en-face electron fields (Figure 1.7)
■ Interactions of photons with matter:
  ■ Coherent scattering: only important in diagnostic x-rays (energy is unchanged, only direction has changed)

TABLE 1.2 Selected Beam Characteristics

Photons	Electrons
^{60}Co: D_{max} = 0.5 cm, attenuation ~5%/cm	MeV/5 = D_{max} (cm)
4 MV: D_{max} = 1.0 cm	MeV/4 = 90% IDL
6 MV: D_{max} = 1.5 cm, attenuation ~4%/cm	MeV/3 = 80% IDL
10 MV: D_{max} = 2.5 cm	MeV/2.33 = 50% IDL
18 MV: D_{max} = 3.5 cm, attenuation ~3%/cm	MeV/2 = R_p

Abbreviations: ^{60}Co, Cobalt 60; IDL, isodose line; R_p, practical range.

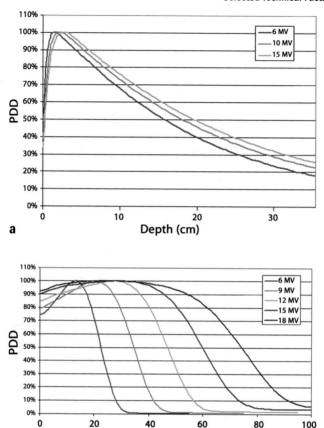

FIGURE 1.4 (a) Photon depth-dose curves, 10×10 cm field, 100 SSD. (b) Electron depth-dose curves, 10×10 cm electron cone, 100 SSD. Note: Surface dose decreases with increasing photon energy and increases with increasing electron energy.

- Photoelectric effect: important at diagnostic energies and useful in improving imaging quality due to increased contrast. Photon in, electron and characteristic x-rays out (probability proportional to Z^3/E^3)
- Compton scattering/incoherent scatter: photon in, electron and photon out (probability proportional to $1/E$, independent of Z, Compton component begins to dominate at energies of ~200 keV)
- Pair production: photon in, electron and positron out (requires 1.02 MeV threshold)

FIGURE 1.5 Posteroanterior beam, 10×10 cm fields, 100 SAD, dose normalized to isocenter placed at a 9-cm depth: (a) 6- and (b) 15-MV photons without heterogeneity correction; (c) 6- and (d) 15-MV photons with heterogeneity correction.

■ Photodisintegration: photon in, neutron or proton out (also known as γ, n or γ, p reaction, requires ~7 MeV threshold)
■ Interactions of electrons with matter:
  ■ Inelastic collision with atomic nucleus: bremsstrahlung
  ■ Inelastic collision with atomic electrons: ionization or excitation
  ■ Elastic collision with atomic nucleus
  ■ Elastic collision with atomic electrons

Important characteristics of electron beams:
  ■ Obliquity should be avoided with electron fields as surface dose increases, penetration decreases, and D_{max} moves toward the surface.

FIGURE 1.6 Anteroposterior/posteroanterior beams, 10×10 cm fields, 100 SAD, dose normalized to midplane: (a) 6- and (b) 15-MV photons without heterogeneity correction; (c) 6- and 15-MV (d) photons with heterogeneity correction.

- Isodose line "bulging" (Figure 1.7):
  - Low-isodose lines bulge out for both high- and low-energy electrons.
  - High-isodose lines constrict for high-energy electrons (not for low-energy electrons).
- Surface dose increases with increasing electron energy due to increased side-scatter.
- X-ray contamination is greater for high-energy electron beams and highest at the beam's central axis (mainly due to bremsstrahlung interactions with the scattering foil).
- The minimum field diameter for an electron beam should be energy/2 (to allow for adequate scatter for dose buildup).

FIGURE 1.7 Isodose distributions of 16- and 9-MeV electrons are compared to emphasize greater constriction of high-isodose lines when using high-energy electron beams.

- DD decreases as field size decreases.
- Proton Radiotherapy
  - The dosimetric properties of protons differ from photons and electrons.
  - Proton DD increases slowly until peaking sharply at a maximum value (Bragg peak) and then quickly falling to zero as opposed to falling off slowly after a short buildup region (Figure 1.8).
  - The depth of the Bragg peak is energy dependent.

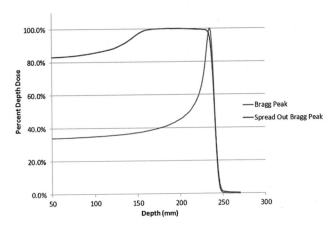

FIGURE 1.8 Percent depth dose curve for a monoenergetic proton beam and the same beam after modulation showing the Spread Out Bragg Peak (SOBP). The width of the SOBP is defined as the distance between the distal and proximal 90% dose positions.

- For clinical use, a monoenergetic proton beam is modulated to introduce protons of several different energies. Thus the sharp Bragg peak widens into a Spread Out Bragg Peak (SOBP). By choosing proton energies relative to the depth of the tumor, the SOBP can be designed to cover the PTV very conformally.
- The steep falloff of dose following the Bragg peak to zero means that exit dose from a proton beam is dramatically less than that of an X-ray beam.
- Proton beams are not shaped with an MLC as in a photon beam, but rather by using specially milled compensators.
- The fundamentals of treatment planning remain the same for protons as they do for photons and electrons.

SELECTED BRACHYTHERAPY FACTS

- Isotope properties (Table 1.3)
- Principles of decay
  - Decay constant (λ): fraction decaying/unit time = 0.693/half-life
  - Half-life = 0.693/decay constant
  - Current activity = Initial activity $\times$ e$^{(-\lambda \times time)}$
- Rules of thumb regarding decay:
  - Amount remaining: 10% remains after 3.3 half-lives, 1% after 6.6 half-lives, 0.1% after 10 half-lives
  - Cs-137: approximately 2.3% decay per year
  - Co-60: approximately 1% decay per month
  - I-125 and Ir-192: approximately 1% decay per day
  - Pd-103: approximately 4% decay per day

ICRU 38 "Dose and Volume Specification for Reporting Intracavitary Therapy in Gynecology"

- Low dose rates (LDR), between 0.4 and 2 Gy/h; high dose rates (HDR), >12 Gy/h
- Bladder reference point:
  - Foley catheter is inserted and the balloon filled with 7-cm^3 radio-opaque contrast fluid. Tension is applied to bring catheter against the urethra.
  - Lateral radiograph: posterior surface of the balloon on an AP line drawn through the center of the balloon.
  - AP radiograph: center of the balloon.

TABLE 1.3 Isotopes

Radionuclide	Decay	Beta Energy
Pd-103	Electron Capture	None
I-125	Electron Capture	None
Ir-192	Gamma	240-670 keV
Au-198	Gamma	0.96 MeV (max)
Cs-137	Gamma	0.514-1.17 MeV
Ra-226	Gamma	0.017-3.26 MeV
Co-60	Gamma	313 keV (max)
I-131	Beta	791 keV (max); 180 keV (avg)
Sr-89	Beta	1.46 MeV (max); 583 keV (avg)
P-32	Beta	1.7 MeV (max); 695 keV (avg)
Y-90	Beta	2.282 MeV (max); 937 keV (avg)
Ru-106	Beta	3.54 MeV (max)
Sm-153	Mixed	233 keV (avg)

Abbreviations: avg, average; Au, gold; Co, cobalt; Cs, cesium; I, iodine; Ir, iridium;
P, phosphorus; Pd, palladium; Ra, radium; Ru, ruthenium; Sm, samarium; Sr, strontium;
Y, yttrium.
*Exposure rate constant in R cm^2/h mCi except for radium and radon (R cm^2/h mg).

■ Rectal reference point:
  ■ Visualize posterior vaginal wall with opacification of the vaginal cavity with radio-opaque gauze used for packing.
  ■ Lateral radiograph: an AP line is drawn from the lower end of the intra-uterine source (or the middle of the intravaginal source). Reference point is on this line, 5 mm behind posterior vaginal wall.
  ■ AP radiograph: the reference point is at the lower end of the intrauterine source (or the middle of the intravaginal source).

Gamma Energy	Half-Life	Exposure Rate Constant*	Lead HVL (mm)
21 keV (avg)	17 d	1.48	0.008
28 keV (avg)	60.2 d	1.46	0.025
380 keV (avg)	74.2 d	4.69	2.5
412 keV	2.7 d	2.38	2.5
662 keV (max)	30 y	3.26	5.5
830 keV (avg)	1622 y	8.25	12
1.25 MeV (avg)	5.26 y	13.07	11
80-637 keV	8 d	2.2	3
–	50.5 d	–	–
–	14.3 d	–	0.1
–	64 h	–	–
–	366 d	–	–
103 keV (avg)	1.93 d		

REFERENCE

1. Ellis RE. The distribution of active bone marrow in the adult. *Phys Med Biol* 1961;5:255–258.

2   Tools for Simulation and Treatment

Neil M. Woody and Gregory M. M. Videtic

TECHNIQUES IN POSITIONING AND IMMOBILIZATION

Thermoplastic Mesh

- Thermoplastic mesh is a polymer that becomes soft and flexible when heated in a water bath, providing a customizable material for reproducible immobilization.
- Thermoplastic mesh is commonly used for immobilizing the head but may be used at other sites such as the abdomen or extremities.
- Three-point masks (Figure 2.1a) are commonly used for brain and head and neck treatments.
- Bolus material may be held to the region of interest with the use of a swimmer's cap under a thermoplastic mesh mask (Figure 2.1b).

FIGURE 2.1 (a) Patient with a three-point thermoplastic mask (points superior and lateral to head fixed to table). (b) Swimmer's cap holding tissue-equivalent bolus material in place.

FIGURE 2.2 Patient with five-point thermoplastic mask (points superior, lateral to head, and shoulders fixed to table).

- Five-point masks (Figure 2.2) provide additional immobilization of the shoulders and are particularly useful for low-neck and stereotactic treatments.
- Body molds (Figure 2.3) may be created for immobilization in abdominal and pelvic treatments.

Cradle-Type Devices

- Molds occupying the space between the treatment table and the patient can be custom-made to provide a reproducible positioning system.
- Common materials include foam (Alpha cradle) and vacuum-locking beads in airtight bags (eg, Elekta BodyFIX, Stockholm, Sweden). Patients are placed in the cradle, and vacuum suction is applied, locking the beads in place.
- Partial-body cradles are used for immobilization of a portion of the body, for example, an extremity (Figure 2.4a).

FIGURE 2.3 Thermoplastic body mold.

FIGURE 2.4 (a) Woman with sarcoma of the left arm, immobilized in a partial-body vacuum-locking bag. (b) Woman with sarcoma of the left leg, immobilized prone in a full-body vacuum-locking bag.

- Full-body cradles are used for stereotactic treatments and when immobilization at multiple points is desired (Figure 2.4b).

Modular Systems

- Modular systems exist for custom immobilization of nearly every body site; an example is shown in Figure 2.5a and b.
- Custom adjustments can be made via modules to position the head, arms, chest, abdomen, pelvis, and legs.
- Prone position on "Belly board" systems allows space for anterior displacement of abdominal contents (Figure 2.5c).

Stereotactic Systems

- BodyFIX with total body cover sheet
  - A full-body vacuum-locking (vac-loc) bag (BodyFIX) beneath the patient is combined with a thin plastic sheet that covers the patient. The thin plastic sheet is attached to the vac-loc bag by an adhesive film at the edges. Vacuum suction is applied to remove air between the thin plastic sheet and the vac-loc bag to further limit patient motion (Figure 2.6).

FIGURE 2.5 Modular positioning system for (a) upper- and (b) lower-body positioning. Also shown is a belly board for anterior displacement of bowel (c).

Breath Control Systems

- Abdominal compression
  - An adjustable paddle placed in the epigastric region or a belt placed at the level of the umbilicus is adjusted to restrict breathing to a tolerable level that minimizes target motion (Figure 2.7).
  - Choice of paddle or belt depends on target location; less interference occurs using a belt for patients with inferiorly located chest lesions.

FIGURE 2.6 Patient positioned supine in a full-body vacuum locking bag. A vacuum-sealed total-body cover sheet is covering the patient to provide additional immobilization. Adhesive attachments for infrared markers are present on the cover sheet.

FIGURE 2.7 Patient positioned supine with arms above the head using a combined modular arm immobilization system and a full-body vacuum-locking bag. Abdominal compression is applied with an adjustable paddle to restrict tumor motion. A bellows system is placed to track respiratory phase for 4D-CT. Infrared markers are part of the image-guided radiation therapy verification system for use at the time of treatment.

- Breath control
  - Breath-holding techniques, such as active breathing control, often use valves to control airflow through a mouthpiece. The breath hold is conducted during simulation and replicated at the time of treatment.
- Chairs
  - Patients in distress who cannot lie flat or recline may, in emergency situations, be treated in the sitting position using a suitably designed chair providing stability and a reference system.

TECHNIQUES IN SIMULATION

- 2-Dimensional (fluoroscopy)
  - Fluoroscopy is used to position the patient based on disease, bony land marks, and radiopaque wires placed by the physician.
  - Radiographs are made to include the entire treatment volume, from which custom blocks may be designed to avoid normal tissues.
- 3-Dimensional (Computed Tomography [CT]) (3DCT)
  - Conventional CT images are acquired.
  - The isocenter is placed within the tumor volume (at least D_{max} from the surface).

- Marks are placed on the patient for triangulation to the isocenter.
- Shifts from this isocenter may be made at the time of treatment planning.
- Allows for planning based on 3D volumes, creation of beam's-eye view, and highly conformal planning, both forward and inverse.
- 4-Dimensional (4D-CT)
  - Allows for visualization of target and organ motion.
  - Computed tomography image sets are acquired over consecutive breathing cycles. They are sorted for viewing by respiratory phase detected by a fiducial system and/or a device to record the respiratory cycle, for example, Varian (Palo Alto, CA), RPM, and Philips (Andover, MA) abdominal bellows device (Figure 2.7).
- Contouring volumes
  - The advent of computer treatment planning systems using 3D and 4D imaging has allowed for physicians to create "volumes" that represent target and normal structures.
  - The Radiation Therapy Oncology Group (RTOG) has made numerous atlases available to aid in contouring volumes (www.rtog.org/CoreLab/ContouringAtlases.aspx).
  - Secondary image sets can be coregistered with simulation CT images to aid in volume localization (eg, magnetic resonance imaging [MRI], positron emission tomography [PET], Magnetic Resonance Spectroscopy [MRS], and angiogram).
  - 4D-CT may be reconstructed as phases of the breathing cycle or as maximal intensity projection (MIP) to a display of maximal extent of motion of a structure over the respiratory cycle.

TECHNIQUES IN LOCALIZATION AT THE TIME OF TREATMENT DELIVERY

Gaiting

- Gaiting techniques coordinate the timing of radiation beam "on time" with a desired target position, as determined by a reference fiducial system.
  - For example, beam on within a selected phase of the respiratory cycle (eg, rest phase of exhalation)
  - Active breathing control represents a form of gaiting wherein the respiratory cycle is held for a period of time by a valve device (Figure 2.8).

Portal Imaging

- Megavoltage radiographs may be taken prior to treatment delivery to confirm patient's positioning.
  - These are recommended to be conducted at least weekly.

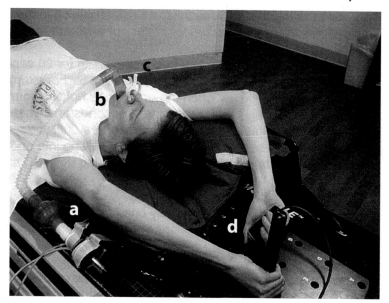

FIGURE 2.8 Active breathing control system with valve (a), mouthpiece (b), nosepiece (c) and patient-controlled valve release (d).

- Orthogonal films (eg, AP and lateral) allow for corrections in patient's position.
- Electronic (digital) portal imaging uses amorphous silicon to create digital portal films.

Image-Guided Radiation Therapy (IGRT)

- IGRT is a method whereby high-precision radiotherapy (RT) is delivered through imaging verification target or reference structure setup prior to treatment.

Methods
- Ultrasound
  - May be referenced to simulation CT or ultrasound conducted at the time of simulation (Figure 2.9)
  - Non-ionizing method to locate target
  - Limited by interuser variability (eg, the amount of pressure applied and the location where the transducer is placed)
  - Most commonly used to locate prostate and prostatic bed; although also used to locate breast tumor bed

FIGURE 2.9 Transabdominal ultrasound in coronal and sagittal planes used for prostate localization for a patient receiving imaged-guided IMRT.

- In-room orthogonal radiographs
  - Mounted to gantry or in ceiling and floor
  - Radiography central axes intersect at the isocenter
  - Uses bony landmark or implanted fiducial markers as a reference point
  - Allows for intrafraction monitoring (ie, imaging while the therapeutic beam is turned on)
- Calypso® beacon transponders
  - Radiofrequency transponders
    • Require implantation
    • Currently only used routinely for prostate radiotherapy (Figure 2.10)
  - Allow for triangulation and intrafraction tracking
- Cone beam and helical imaging
  - Kilovoltage (KV) or MV imaging may be used to locate structures on the day of treatment (Figure 2.11). Alignment may be made to bone or soft tissue.
  - KV radiography tube is mounted either at 90° to the gantry or in line with the gantry.
  - Megavoltage imaging using linear accelerator beam (may be degraded to KV energy to improve resolution). Translating the table during image acquisition provides helical imaging.
  - Volumetric information for understanding of positional errors in the x, y, z, roll, pitch, and yaw directions is given.
- CT on rails
  - Mobile diagnostic-type KV CT scanner in treatment vault.

FIGURE 2.10 AP digitally reconstructed radiograph of a patient with implanted Calypso beacon transponders (green, yellow, and blue); the prostate is outlined in red. The patient also has an urethrogram study.

FIGURE 2.11 KV cone beam CT used for image-guided radiotherapy in a patient with prostate cancer. Axial and coronal images are shown colocalized with the simulation CT.

- CT translates over the patient on a rail system.
- Allows for high-resolution, diagnostic-quality imaging.
- Doses from techniques that use ionizing radiation are in the range of 0.1 cGy for orthogonal KV systems and 1 to 10 cGy per fraction for KV and MV cone beam scans, depending on field size and amount of rotation.

- Treatment tables with 6 degrees of motion freedom (x, y, z, roll, pitch, and yaw) have been developed to compensate for deviations in setup found with image-guided radiation therapy.
- Monitoring of external fiducial markers or light surface projections
  - Infrared markers placed on the patient may be monitored with in-room infrared cameras (see Figure 2.7).
  - 3D surface mapping is emerging as a nonionizing alternative to assist with patient alignment.

3   Central Nervous System Radiotherapy

Abigail L. Stockham, John H. Suh, and Samuel T. Chao

GENERAL PRINCIPLES

- General principles for simulation techniques, dose constraints, and planning principles apply to a range of intracranial tumors.
- Dose prescriptions are informed by patient, tumor, and treatment factors.
- Postoperative radiotherapy is usually started 2 to 4 weeks after resection for malignant disease; benign resected tumors may be treated further from resection.

Localization, Immobilization, and Simulation

- Computed tomography (CT) simulation to delineate gross tumor volume (GTV), clinical target volume (CTV), and planning target volume (PTV).

The patient is positioned supine with arms at the sides.

■ Immobilization is achieved with a thermoplastic mask. Head frame is usually used for single-fraction stereotactic radiosurgery (SRS).

■ Use spiral CT to plan with 2 to 3 mm slice acquisition from the vertex through the midcervical spine. Intravenous (IV) contrast for enhancing lesions may be used to delineate the tumor volume/resection cavity.

■ Magnetic resonance imaging (MRI) simulation may be used to avoid issues of coregistration.

Target Volumes and Organs of Interest Definition

■ GTV: tumor volume or postoperative resection cavity appreciable on radiographic imaging, typically MRI.

■ CTV: includes sites at risk for microscopic disease.

■ PTV: allows for daily variation in setup and varies from institution to institution based on that institution's ability to reproduce treatment positions. Consider tighter margins when using image-guided radiation therapy.

■ Regions of interest are identified and contoured (see Table 3.1).

Treatment Planning

Planning

■ Treatment planning is optimized with MRI co-registration to assist in delineating edema with T2 and fluid attenuation and inversion recovery (FLAIR) images as well as to discern the presence or extent of T1-enhancing lesions.

TABLE 3.1 Maximum Point Doses for Fractionated Radiotherapy and SRS for Intracranial Structures of Interest

Structures of Interest	Maximum Point Dose, Gy	
	Fractionated Radiotherapy	**SRS**
Lenses	7	As low as possible
Retina	45–50	As low as possible
Optic nerves	55	8
Optic chiasm	56	8
Cochlea	55	8–9
Pituitary	45	As low as possible
Brainstem	60	12
Spinal cord	50	10

Abbreviation: SRS, stereotactic radiosurgery.

- MRIs used in treatment planning should be obtained postoperatively within 48 hours to avoid ambiguity regarding residual tumor versus postoperative changes/blood. Timing of MRI for treatment planning purposes for benign processes is less critical.

Options

- Point calculations: primarily used in palliative treatment such as whole-brain EBRT (see Chapter 13).
- 3D conformal radiotherapy: standard coplanar or noncoplanar 3D conformal fields are structured to optimize dose to target areas while minimizing dose to critical structures.
- IMRT: may be used to spare critical structures of the brain/spine for its ability to deliver a highly conformal dose to a target while respecting dose constraints to critical structures.
- Volumetric modulated arc therapy (VMAT): used to effectively increase the number of beam angles and potentially decrease both the total number of monitor units and treatment times for complex brain tumor treatments near critical structures (1).
- Image-guided radiotherapy (IGRT): used for lesions particularly close to critical structures to ensure accurate daily setup; often used with highly conformal radiotherapy (IMRT, fractionated stereotactic radiotherapy, VMAT).

Critical Structures

The brain contains several structures considered to be "serial structures" emphasizing the importance of evaluating point doses in addition to volumetric doses (see Table 3.1).

Single-Fraction SRS

Indications

- Benign and malignant brain tumors, vascular malformations, and functional disorders.
- Single-fraction SRS alone is most appropriate for well-circumscribed targets (≤4 cm in diameter; ≥0.3–0.5 cm from optic apparatus).
- Consider fractionated radiotherapy for tumors too large for SRS or abutting critical structures, especially optic nerve and chiasm.

SRS technique

- Intravenous line placed for midazolam sedation.
- Lidocaine injected at four locations on the scalp for frame placement.
- Image with MRI (1 mm slices) then CT. Coregister scans.

- Planning: volume is T1 enhancing tumor or other anatomic structures for functional disorders.
- Dexamethasone at 6 to 10 mg IV 30 minutes before the procedure (consider continuing dexamethasone for 1 to 2 weeks post-procedure if concerned for edema).

SRS planning goals

- The conformality index, the ratio of the prescription isodose volume divided by the tumor volume, should be ≤2. The homogeneity index, or the ratio of the maximum dose divided by the peripheral dose, should be ≤2.
- PTV is enhancing lesion on T1 MRI with gadolinium. For very superficial lesions bolus may be used, held in place by a swimmer's cap.

GLIOMA—HIGH GRADE

Indications and Options for Treatment

- Adjuvant therapy in the postoperative setting
- Definitive treatment in the inoperable setting

Localization, Immobilization, Simulation for Fractionated Radiotherapy (RT)/Fractionated Stereotactic RT (FSRT)

- Per general principles.

Volumes, Dose, and Fractionation

- Anaplastic astrocytoma
  - Volumes
    - GTV: postoperative T1-weighted MRI contrast enhancement or T2 signal change
    - CTV: GTV + 1.5 to 2 cm
    - PTV: CTV + 0.3 to 0.5 cm
  - Dose and fractionation
    - 50.4 Gy/1.8 Gy/fx to initial field as above
    - Boost 9 Gy/1.8 Gy/fx to the postoperative contrast-enhancing tumor on T1-weighted MRI GTV with a 1.0 cm margin for CTV
- Anaplastic oligodendroglioma
  - Volumes
    - GTV: postoperative T2 MRI changes
    - CTV: GTV + 1.5 to 2 cm
    - PTV: CTV + 0.3 to 0.5 cm
  - Dose and fractionation

- 50.4 Gy/1.8 Gy/fx to initial field as above
- Boost 9 Gy/1.8 Gy/fx to postoperative contrast-enhancing tumor on T1-weighted MRI GTV with a 1.0 cm margin for CTV
  - Glioblastoma (see Figure 3.1)
    - Volumes
      - GTV: postoperative resection cavity, contrast enhancement, or edema on T2/FLAIR
      - CTV: GTV + 2 cm if edema on T2/FLAIR or 2.5 cm if no edema with respect for natural boundaries
      - PTV: CTV + 0.3 to 0.5 cm
  - Dose and fractionation
    - 46 Gy/2 Gy/fx to T2/FLAIR change as above
    - Boost 14 Gy/2 Gy/fx to the resection cavity or postoperative T1 contrast enhancement (GTV) with a 2.0 cm margin for CTV and 0.3 to 0.5 cm PTV

Special Considerations

- Elderly patients or patients with poor performance status may be considered for altered fractionation, including:
- 40 Gy/2.67 Gy/fx
- 37.5 Gy/2.5 Gy/fx
- 30 Gy/3 Gy/fx (as whole-brain RT)

FIGURE 3.1 (a) A 55-year-old man with right parietal glioblastoma (GBM) with spread through the corpus callosum, s/p stereotactic biopsy. GTV based on contrast enhancement in red, and T2/FLAIR changes in green. EBRT: 60 Gy/2 Gy/fx, via 5-field IMRT; 6 MV photons prescribed to the 98% isodose line (IDL); 60 Gy IDL in yellow. (b) Beam arrangement for this patient. Noncoplanar, 5-field plan. T1 contrast enhancement in red, T2/FLAIR in green. *Continued on next page.*

c

FIGURE 3.1 (*Continued*) (c) DVH for this patient. Note: dose constraints adapted to avoid compromising dose to treatment volume. (d) A 31-year-old woman with a left frontoparietal low-grade glioma per stereotactic biopsy. The radiographic enhancement is highly suggestive of high-grade astrocytoma. T2 signal change with a 2 cm margin for CTV and 5 mm margin for PTV in green. T1 contrast enhancement with 1 cm margin for CTV and 5 mm margin for PTV in red. T2 signal change PTV treated to 50.4 Gy followed by a 9 Gy boost to the area of contrast enhancement plus 1 cm margin for CTV and 5 mm margin for PTV.

GLIOMA—LOW GRADE

Indications and Options for Treatment

- Definitive therapy
- Adjuvant therapy in the postoperative setting

Localization, Immobilization, Simulation for Fractionated RT/FSRT

- Per general principles

Volumes, Dose, and Fractionation

- Volumes (see Figure 3.2)

Isodose
60 Gy
54 Gy
36 Gy

FIGURE 3.2 A 22-year-old right-handed man with right temporal low-grade mixed glioma, near-total resection 2.5 years ago, now progression. EBRT alone: 54 Gy/1.8 Gy/fx, via 5-field IMRT, mix 6/10 MV photons prescribed to the 97% IDL. T2 signal change in red, PTV in green = GTV + 2 cm (CTV), then + 0.3 cm (PTV). 54 Gy IDL in yellow.

- GTV: signal change on T2 MRI
- CTV: GTV + 1.5 to 2 cm
- PTV: CTV + 0.5 cm
- Dose and fractionation
  - 54 Gy/1.8 Gy/fx

Special Considerations

- Treat gemistocytic astrocytoma as per anaplastic astrocytoma.

BRAINSTEM GLIOMA

Indications for Treatment

- Radiotherapy is standard treatment for inoperable brainstem glioma.
- Lesions are usually not biopsied.

Localization, Immobilization, Simulation for Fractionated RT/FSRT

- Per general principles

Volumes, Dose, and Fractionation

- Volumes (see Figure 3.3)
  - GTV: greatest dimension on T1 or T2 MRI
  - CTV: GTV + 2 cm margin with respect for natural boundaries
  - PTV: CTV + 0.3 to 0.5 cm margin with respect for natural boundaries
- Dose and fractionation
  - 54 Gy/1.8 Gy/fx
  - 50.4 Gy/1.8 Gy/fx

FIGURE 3.3 A 21-year-old woman with brain stem low-grade oligodendroglioma, 1p19q intact, status post biopsy. GTV in red by all MRI sequences. PTV in blue (GTV + 2 cm margin; + 0.3 cm margin for PTV). EBRT: 54 Gy/1.8 Gy/fx, via 7-field IMRT with 6 MV photons prescribed to 100% IDL.

MENINGIOMA

Indications for Treatment

- Benign: inoperability, subtotal resection, recurrence
- Atypical: inoperability, status post gross total resection, status post subtotal resection
- Malignant: inoperability, status post gross total resection, status post subtotal resection

Localization, Immobilization, Simulation for Fractionated RT/FSRT

- Per general principles

Volumes, Dose, and Fractionation

- Volumes (see Figure 3.4a)
  - GTV: enhancement on T1 MRI
  - CTV: GTV = CTV
    - Consider 0.5 cm CTV for recurrent disease or no MRI coregistration
  - PTV: CTV + 0.3 to 0.5 cm
- Dose and fractionation (definitive)
  - Benign: 54 Gy/1.8 Gy/fx
    - GTV: enhancement on T1 MRI
    - CTV: GTV = CTV
    - PTV: CTV + 0.3 to 0.5 cm
  - Atypical: 59.4 Gy/1.8 Gy/fx
    - GTV: enhancement on T1 MRI
    - CTV: GTV + 1 cm with respect for natural barriers
    - PTV: CTV + 0.3 to 0.5 cm

- Malignant: 59.4 to 60 Gy/1.8 to 2 Gy/fx
  - GTV: enhancement on T1 MRI
  - CTV: GTV + 2 cm with respect for natural barriers
  - PTV: CTV + 0.3 to 0.5 cm
- Dose and fractionation (postoperative)
  - Benign: 54 Gy/1.8 Gy/fx for subtotal resection
    - GTV: enhancement on T1 MRI
    - CTV: GTV = CTV
    - PTV: CTV + 0.3 to 0.5 cm
  - Atypical: 54 Gy/1.8 Gy/fx for gross total resection and 59.4 Gy/1.8 Gy/fx for subtotal resection
    - GTV: enhancement on T1 MRI
    - CTV: GTV + 1 cm with respect for natural barriers

FIGURE 3.4 (a) A 53-year-old woman with left cavernous sinus meningioma. On axial and coronal images, GTV (area of contrast enhancement) in red. EBRT: 54 Gy/1.8 Gy/fx, via 7-field IMRT with 6 MV photons prescribed to the 100% IDL. (b) A 40-year-old woman with left tentorial meningioma with brainstem compression, status post subtotal resection treated with Gamma Knife® (GK) SRS, 12 Gy prescribed to the 50% IDL, seen in yellow.

- PTV: CTV + 0.3 to 0.5 cm
- Malignant: 59.4 to 60 Gy /1.8 to 2 Gy/fx for both gross and subtotal resections
  - GTV: enhancement on T1 MRI
  - CTV: GTV + 2 cm with respect for natural barriers
  - PTV: CTV + 0.3 to 0.5 cm
- SRS (see Figure 3.4b) may be used if:
  - The lesion is more than 0.3 to 0.5 cm away from the optic chiasm.
  - The dose is 13 to 14 Gy (higher doses may be considered for atypical and malignant meningiomas).
  - Optic chiasm dose is limited to 8 to 9 Gy with consideration that some institutions accept higher doses to the optic chiasm.

Special Considerations

- Inclusion of dural tail is controversial, particularly with regard to SRS.
- Care must be taken for parasagittal lesions, as malignant edema may occur with treatment of parasagittal meningiomas.

PITUITARY ADENOMA

Indications for Treatment

- Unresectable or subtotally resected lesions
- SRS is the preferred treatment modality.

Localization, Immobilization, Simulation for Fractionated RT/FSRT

- Per general principles

Volumes, Dose, and Fractionation

Fractionated radiotherapy

- Volumes (see Figure 3.5)
  - GTV: gadolinium enhancement on T1 MRI with contrast
  - CTV: GTV = CTV
  - Consider 0.5 cm CTV for recurrent disease or no MRI coregistration
  - PTV: CTV + 0.5 cm
- Dose and fractionation
  - 45 Gy/1.8 Gy/fx for nonfunctional pituitary adenoma and 50.4 Gy/1.8 Gy/fx for secretory adenomas
- SRS
  - Preferred treatment modality
  - Feasible if lesion is more than 0.3 to 0.5 cm away from the optic chiasm.

FIGURE 3.5 A 61-year-old woman with nonsecreting pituitary macroadenoma, status-post transsphenoidal resection 14 years prior to recurrence. Recurrence treated with subtotal transsphenoidal re-resection followed by 45 Gy/1.8 Gy/fx IMRT, via an 8-field technique with 6 MV photons prescribed to the 100% IDL.

- Dose
  - 15 to 16 Gy for nonfunctional adenomas
  - 18 to 25 Gy for secretory adenomas

VESTIBULAR SCHWANNOMA

Indications for Radiotherapy Treatment

- To maintain hearing
- Radiographic progression

Localization, Immobilization, Simulation for Fractionated RT/FSRT

- Per general principles

Volumes, Dose, and Fractionation

- Volumes (see Figure 3.4)
  - GTV: T1-weighted enhancing tumor
  - CTV: GTV = CTV
  - Consider 0.5 cm CTV for recurrent disease or no MRI co-registration
  - PTV: CTV + 0.5 cm for fractionated EBRT, PTV = CTV for SRS
  - Contour applicable regions of interest as seen in Table 3.1

- Dose (see Figure 3.6)
  - 45 to 54 Gy/1.8 Gy/fx
  - SRS dose 13 Gy to 50% IDL with gamma knife SRS (Figure 3.6) and 80% IDL with linear accelerator (LINAC) SRS
- Fractionation
  - Fractionated EBRT or FSRT for tumors 3.5 cm or normal/minimal hearing loss and SRS for lesions smaller than 3.5 cm

Special Considerations

- Patients with neurofibromatosis-2 are often affected by bilateral vestibular schwannomas (synchronously or metachronously), increasing the risk for bilateral deafness.
- Consider fractionated EBRT, as it may allow greater hearing preservation than SRS.

FIGURE 3.6 Left vestibular schwannoma with classic "ice cream cone" shape. Treated with GK SRS, 13 Gy to the 50% IDL. Yellow: 50% IDL; green: 100% IDL.

ARTERIOVENOUS MALFORMATION

Indications and Options for Treatment

- Reduce the risk of hemorrhage and neurologic deficits/symptoms.
- Spetzler-Martin I and II—surgical intervention preferred for faster decline of risk of hemorrhage.
- Spetzler-Martin grade III—surgical intervention versus SRS with consideration for factors included in Spetzler-Martin grading system (size, eloquence, and venous drainage) as they apply to an individual case.
- Spetzler-Martin grade IV/V—staged radiosurgery with multiple isocenters may be feasible for select large lesions (2).

Localization, Immobilization, Simulation

- Per general principles

Volumes, Dose, and Fractionation

- Volume
  - As delineated on high-volume MRI and angiogram
- Dose
  - 14 to 27 Gy

Special Considerations

- Aneurysms on feeding arteries of arteriovenous malformations must be addressed prior to interventions on the arteriovenous malformation nidus to avoid increased arterial pressure at the site of aneurysm following arteriovenous malformation nidus ablation.

SPINAL CORD TUMORS

Indications and Options for Treatment

- Adjuvant or definitive treatment.
- In the setting of inoperability or low-grade gliomas, particularly in young children, it is reasonable to attempt to delay radiotherapy as long as is feasible.

Localization, Immobilization, Simulation for Fractionated RT/FSRT

- Positioning: supine with arms at the side
- Localization: coregister planning CT with preoperative T1 and T2 MRI to delineate GTV.
- Immobilization: vacuum bag device

TABLE 3.2 Approaches to Spinal Cord Tumors

Histology	Surgery	Adjuvant Treatment
Low-grade astrocytoma (WHO I-II)	Attempt GTR (mostly obtained with pilocytic astro)	GTR: none STR/Biopsy (Bx): focal EBRT to 50. 4–54 Gy
High-grade astrocytoma (WHO III-IV)	Bx or STR (difficult to resect because of infiltrative nature)	Focal RT to 50.4 Gy (CTV) with boost to 54.0–59.4 (GTV), consider chemotherapy
Meningioma	Attempt GTR	GTR: none STR/Bx: observation (low grade [LG]) vs. focal EBRT to 54 Gy
Schwannoma/ neurofibroma	Attempt GTR (frequently need to sacrifice nerve)	GTR: none STR/Bx: 50.4–54.0 Gy /1.8 Gy/fx. Consider SRS for skull base (Florida)
Hemangioma	GTR (for cord compression)	GTR: none None (or failed embolization, ethanol injection, vertebroplasty), symptomatic: focal EBRT to 40 Gy at 2 Gy/fx
Spinal canal (ie, neurofibrosarcoma/ malignant peripheral nerve sheath tumor (MPNST)	Attempt GTR (infrequently obtained)	Charged particles to 60–70 Gy +/- chemotherapy. Consider IMRT
Vertebral body (ie, chondrosarcoma, chordoma, osteogenic sarcoma)	Attempt GTR (infrequently obtained)	Charged particles to 70–78 Gy postoperative +/-chemotherapy. Consider IMRT. Consider protons

- Simulation: high-resolution CT scan with or without IV contrast.
  - For lesions located in the superior spine, the cerebellum should be included through at least two vertebrae inferior to the lesion.
  - For lesions located in the inferior spine, the entire sacrum should be included through at least two vertebrae superior to the lesion.

Planning

- For spinal cord tumors, contour normal structures in the treatment field and follow dose constraints as per tolerances described for definitive treatment in that body area (eg, thorax, abdomen, pelvis).

Volumes, Dose, and Fractionation

- Low-grade gliomas:
  - GTV: preoperative signal change on T2 MRI
  - CTV: GTV + 0.5 to 1 cm cephalad/caudad with radial margins to include nerve roots
  - PTV: CTV + 0.3 to 0.5 cm
- High-grade gliomas (Table 3.2):
  - GTV: preoperative enhancing volume on T1 gadolinium contrasted MRI
  - CTV: GTV + 1.5 cm cephalad/caudad with radial margins to include nerve roots
  - PTV: CTV + 0.3 to 0.5 cm
- Include cyst or syrinx volumes in GTV if involved by tumor.
- CSI for grossly disseminated disease.

REFERENCES

1. Davidson MT, Masucci GL, Follwell M, et al. Single arc volumetric modulated arc therapy for complex brain gliomas: is there an advantage as compared to intensity modulated radiotherapy or by adding a partial arc? *Technol Cancer Res Treat.* 2012;11(3):211–220.

2. Spetzler RF, Martin NA. A proposed grading system for arteriovenous malformations. *J Neurosurg.* 1986;65:476–483.

4   Head and Neck Radiotherapy

*Aryavarta M. S. Kumar, John F. Greskovich, Jr,
and Shlomo A. Koyfman*

GENERAL PRINCIPLES

- Radical radiotherapy is indicated either in the primary management of head and neck (H&N) cancer (with concurrent chemotherapy for locally advanced disease) or in the postoperative setting (+/− concurrent chemotherapy) if there are high-risk features (eg, T3/4, N2/3, + perineural invasion [PNI], + lymphovascular space invasion [LVSI], close/+ margins, + extracapsular extension [ECE], recurrent disease).

RADIOTHERAPY

Localization, Immobilization, and Simulation

- Historically, 2D simulation and field delineation were based on anatomic landmarks.
- CT-based volumetric treatment planning of gross tumor volume (GTV), clinical target volume (CTV), and planning target volume (PTV).
- Patient position is generally supine with arms at sides, shoulders relaxed downward, and neck neutral or extended.
- Immobilization involves 3-point thermoplastic head mask; 5-point head and shoulder mask preferred for intensity-modulated radiation therapy (IMRT).
  - Tongue depressor (aka, intraoral stent) helps stabilize tongue and separate palate from the tongue.
  - Consider coaching patients to not swallow while the beam is on to avoid tongue/larynx motion, especially for 3D boost fields or IMRT.
- Contiguous 3 mm spiral computed tomography (CT) slices are acquired from the top of the brain through the upper mediastinum.
- Intravenous (IV) contrast is preferred to delineate major blood vessels.
- A positron emission tomography (PET) scan is recommended in delineating the GTV
  - Some studies suggest that PET may decrease the primary GTV by 10% to 50% and increase the nodal GTV by identifying lymph node (LN) as negative by CT criteria (1).

Target Volumes and Organs of Interest Definition

- Reference should be made to the 1993 International Commission on Radiation Units & Measurements (ICRU) report no. 62 for complete description of various target volume definitions (GTV, CTV, and PTV).
- GTV: gross tumor defined by clinical examination and radiographic studies of the primary site and involved lymph nodes (LN) (abnormal LN by CT criteria: >1 cm in short axis or central necrosis). PET fusion is frequently used to guide volume design.
- CTV: consider the extent of local tumor extension and site-specific patterns of spread.
- PTV: accounts for daily setup error and organ motion. Be mindful of anatomic changes during the course of treatment (eg, tumor shrinkage and weight loss).
- Normal anatomy to be routinely identified.
  - Spinal cord (top C1 through T4/5)
  - Glottic larynx
  - Brachial plexus (especially in presence of low-lying neck disease)
  - Mandible

- Normal anatomy to be identified when treating the base of the skull
  - Brainstem
  - Optic nerves/chiasm
  - Eyes
  - Lenses
  - Pituitary gland
  - Middle/inner ears (or cochlea)
- Additional normal anatomy to be identified when using IMRT
  - Parotid glands
  - Submandibular glands
  - Oral cavity
  - Lips
  - Skin (in region of target volumes)
  - Cervical esophagus
  - All unidentified tissue
- Optional normal anatomy that may be identified
  - Uninvolved pharyngeal constrictor muscles (aka, OAR pharynx)

Treatment Planning—Definitive Radiotherapy

External beam therapy

- IMRT
  - Standard of care for definitive treatment of H&N malignancies (except for early-stage glottic cancer) and has mostly replaced 3-field conventional RT technique.
  - Nomenclature: many ways to refer to the final volumes
- The CTV/PTV expansion of the GTV may be called:
  - CTV1/PTV1
  - CTV-high dose (CTV_{HD})/PTV-high dose (PTV_{HD})
  - High-risk CTV/high-risk PTV
  - CTV_{dose}/ PTV_{dose}, eg, CTV_{70}/PTV_{70}
- The CTV/PTV, including elective/low-risk nodes, can be called:
  - CTV2/PTV2
  - CTV-elective dose (CTV_{ED})/PTV-elective dose (PTV_{ED})
  - Low-risk CTV/low-risk PTV
  - CTV_{dose}/ PTV_{dose}, eg, $CTV_{59.4}$/$PTV_{59.4}$
- The CTV/PTV expansion of the intermediate risk used in some plans can be called:
  - CTV_{INT} /PTV_{INT}
  - CTV_{dose}/ PTV_{dose}, eg, CTV_{63}/PTV_{63}
- Technique: use principles outlined above to identify areas at risk and the appropriate risk-matched dose (involved vs. elective; Figure 4.1a and b)

FIGURE 4.1 A 66-year-old man with cT3N2c squamous cell carcinoma (SCC) of the L tonsil treated with definitive chemoradiation using IMRT. (a) Axial CT slice and (b) coronal CT slice both showing PTV1 (red volume), PTV2 (blue volume), and parotid sparing (dark yellow structure). (c) DVH of treatment plan.

■ Definition of the GTV: as above
■ Definition of the CTV_{HD}: GTV + 3 to 5 mm. Can be reduced to 1 mm when abutting critical normal tissues (eg, tumor invading clivus and abutting brainstem).
■ Definition of CTV_{ED}: all clinically negative, elective nodal areas felt to be at risk of microscopic tumor involvement plus an additional 5 to 10 mm margin around CTV_{HD}. See Radiation Therapy Oncology Group (RTOG) atlas for delineation of nodal stations (note: atlas developed for N0 patients; www.rtog.org/CoreLab/ContouringAtlases/HNAtlases .aspx).

■ Definition of the CTV_{INT}: if GTV margin is ill-defined (infiltrative tumor), one may consider an intermediate dose to a 10 mm margin of tissue surrounding selective areas of CTV_{HD}.

■ Definition of the PTV: uniform expansion around CTV. CTV + 5 mm (without image-guided radiotherapy [IGRT]); CTV + 2.5 mm (with IGRT).

■ 3-field approach: currently used to start patient urgently when IMRT plan cannot be developed in a short time. In general, opposed laterals are matched to an anterior supraclavicular (SCV) field to cover primary site and cervical/SCV LN at risk.

Standard lateral field borders (Figure 4.2a)

■ Superior: mastoid tip to cover level II, or the base of the skull, to cover retropharyngeal nodes when indicated.

■ Inferior: above the arytenoids when the larynx is not involved; if the larynx cannot be spared, place the inferior border below the cricoid (or as low as shoulders permit).

■ Anterior: 2 to 3 cm anterior to the tumor, or enough to cover Ib nodes when indicated (anterior border of ramus of mandible).

  ■ Spare small strip of skin anteriorly (below mandibular area) unless tumor extends to subcutaneous tissue or there are large submandibular/jugular LN.

■ Posterior: behind spinous process of C2 when covering level V or at the posterior edge of the vertebral body (off cord) when level V is not included in the field.

  ■ Move posterior border "off cord" to mid-vertebral body at 42 to 44 Gy.

  ■ Supplement blocked portion of off-cord field with posterior en face electrons.

Posterior en-face electron field (aka "post strips")

■ Superior, posterior, inferior: same as initial lateral fields (or may add 5 to 10 mm to account for "bowing in" of high isodose lines with electrons)

■ Anterior

  ■ Abutting posterior border of off-cord field ("hot match")—confirm light fields

  ■ Alternatively, may leave 2 to 3 mm gap to avoid hotspot if lymphatics are adequately covered at depth as per plan

Standard anteroposterior (AP) field borders (Figure 4.2b)

■ Superior: matched to the inferior border of lateral fields

■ Inferior: 1 cm below the clavicles

■ Lateral: cover medial two-thirds of the clavicle

■ Blocks: include a larynx block throughout treatment when not at risk. Include full midline (spinal cord) block if treating AP field above 50 Gy. When the

FIGURE 4.2 A 62-year-old man with cT3N2a squamous cell carcinoma (SCC) of the R base of the tongue for definitive chemoradiation. (a) Digital reconstructed radiograph (DRR) of the lateral field. Purple denotes the original field, green denotes the off-cord field, blue denotes cone down no. 1, and red denotes final cone down. (b) DRR of the anteroposterior low-neck field. Larynx block is in place throughout treatment.

larynx block is contraindicated, consider 0.5 to 1 cm cord block on the lateral field to avoid excessive spinal cord dose from field overlap. If a single isocentric technique used, this block may be omitted.

Boost field borders
- Primary site dependent
- Treat tumor + 1 to 2 cm margin with opposed lateral or oblique fields.
- Enlarged LN can be treated with an appositional electron beam field or opposed oblique (off-cord) fields if neck dissection is not planned.

Optional cone down no. 1 borders (for intermediate risk areas)
- Consider for infiltrative lesions with ill-defined borders to ensure adequate coverage of subclinical disease.
- Cover primary tumor with expanded margins (1.5–2 cm) prior to final cone down.

Brachytherapy
- Historically used for oral cavity lesions, base of tongue (BOT) or nasopharyngeal boost, and recurrent disease.
  - Target is identified (mark before external beam in case of regression) and implant is designed.
  - Single-plane implant for smaller lesions <5 to 10 mm in width. Double-plane implant for 10 to 20 mm lesions. Volumetric implant for anything bigger or irregularly shaped.
  - Needle spacing is typically 10 mm.

Treatment Planning—Postoperative Radiotherapy

- The guiding principles and field design are similar to the definitive setting, with the exception of the lack of a GTV.
- In general, the CTV encompasses the primary tumor bed (based on preoperative imaging, preoperative physical examination and endoscopy, and operative and pathologic findings), any pathologically involved nodal stations, and elective nodal stations, when clinically indicated (Figure 4.3). Consider treating elective areas to lower dose (CTV_{ED}), and boosting areas at very high risk (eg, + margins).

FIGURE 4.3 A 68-year-old man with pT2N0M0 SCC of the oral tongue s/p partial glossectomy (2.2 cm, +PNI, 10 mm depth of invasion (DOI), - lymphovascular invasion (LVSI), -margins, 0/22 LNs). (a) Axial and (b) coronal CT slices showing dose distribution, PTV1 (shaded red), PTV2 (shaded blue). (c) DVH of treatment plan.

Dose/Fractionation

Definitive (chemo)radiotherapy setting

■ IMRT technique (Table 4.1)

When using IMRT, one can alternatively treat primary, upper, and lower neck using a single IMRT plan with appropriate laryngeal constraints (mean dose <45 Gy, if possible).

■ Once-daily fractionation (total doses assume 2 Gy/fx):
  ■ 50 to 54 Gy to elective nodal areas.
  ■ Off-cord field at 42 Gy using photon fields anterior to cord and en face electrons to posterior cervical nodal chain to a dose of 50 to 54 Gy.
  ■ Consider optional cone down no. 1 to 64 Gy for tumors with ill-defined margins.
  ■ Boost GTV to 70 to 74 Gy.

■ Twice-daily fractionation
  ■ 55.2 Gy/1.2 Gy/fx to elective nodal areas.
  ■ Off-cord field at 43.2 Gy using photon fields anterior to cord and en face electrons to posterior cervical nodal chain to dose of 55.2 Gy.
  ■ Consider optional cone down no. 1 to 64.8 Gy/1.2 Gy/fx for tumors with ill-defined margins.
  ■ Boost GTV to 74.4 to 76.8 Gy at 1.2 Gy/fx.
  ■ Treat with at least a 6-hour interfraction interval.

■ Concomitant boost technique (per RTOG 0522)
  ■ 54 Gy at 1.8 Gy/fx to elective nodal areas.
  ■ Off-cord field at 41.4 Gy using photon fields anterior to cord and en face electrons to posterior cervical nodal chain.
  ■ At least 50.4 Gy to 3 cm depth of the posterior neck (when clinically negative) delivered with posterior en face electrons.

TABLE 4.1 IMRT Technique

Per RTOG 1016 (6 Fractions Weekly*)	Per RTOG 0615 (5 Fractions Weekly)
Sites: oropharynx, hypopharynx, larynx	Site: nasopharynx
PTV_{HD} treated to 70 Gy at 2 Gy/fx	PTV_{70} treated to 70 Gy at 2.12 Gy/fx
PTV_{ED} treated to 56 Gy at 1.6 Gy/fx	$PTV_{59.4}$ treated to 59.4 Gy at 1.8 Gy/fx
PTV_{INT} (optional), 59.5–63 Gy at 1.7–1.8 Gy/fx	PTV_{63} (optional), 63 Gy at 1.9 Gy/fx

*Typically with 2 fractions one day per week with at least 6 hour interfraction interval

- At 32.4 Gy, begin concomitant boost to GTV and involved nodes with 1.5 Gy/fx as a second daily fraction for the final 12 treatment days (18 Gy); total dose is 72 Gy.
- Consider optional cone down no. 1 by delivering 1.5 Gy in 6 fx to dose of 63 Gy prior to final cone down.
- Treat with at least a 6-hour interfraction interval.
- Low neck can be treated using a matched anterior field to 50 to 50.4 Gy at 1.8 to 2 Gy/fx delivered to a 3 cm depth when clinically uninvolved. If low neck has gross disease, can deliver 69 to 72 Gy if able to limit brachial plexus to ≤60 Gy. Otherwise, treat to 60 Gy with planned neck dissection, regardless of response (See discussion under "IMRT: Field Matching Techniques" section).

Postoperative setting
- 60 Gy to tumor bed and involved nodes and 56 Gy to elective nodes.
- Consider boosting high-risk areas (known ECE and/or microscopically positive margins) to 66 Gy.

Critical Structures (in Descending Planning Importance; Table 4.2)

Technical factors
- 3D conformal radiotherapy (3DCRT)
  - Doses are calculated *with* heterogeneity corrections.
- IMRT
- Planning goals
  - At least 95% of the PTV receives the prescribed dose (V100 ≥95%).
  - At least 99% of the PTV should receive greater than 93% of the prescribed dose (V93 ≥99%).
  - No more than 1 cc of PTV will receive >110% of prescribed dose.
  - No more than 0.03 cc of PTV should be <9% of prescribed dose.
- Field matching considerations: for lesions above the larynx, can match IMRT field to conventional low anterior neck field or can use a single IMRT plan.
  - Advantage to single IMRT field is the lack of hot/cold spots at the junction (can be up to 20%), but with less laryngeal shielding.
  - Matched fields have better laryngeal shielding and may improve IMRT plan to primary tumor region, but at the expense of junction changes and significant risk of hot/cold spots at match line.
  - To accomplish IMRT/AP field match, use a *half-beam block (monoisocentric technique)*. Close inferior jaw to the central axis for IMRT field and vice versa for the AP field. Feathering the junction superior/inferior 3 mm, twice during treatment, is recommended to reduce hot/cold spots at the junction.

TABLE 4.2 Critical Structures (in Descending Planning Importance)

Spinal cord	PRV (cord + 5 mm) 50 Gy to <0.03 cc
Brainstem PRV (brainstem + 3 mm)	52 Gy to <0.03 cc
Brainstem PRV (BOS)*	<1% to exceed 60 Gy
Optic chiasm/nerves	50 Gy max dose
Optic apparatus PRV (BOS)*	54 Gy max dose
Brachial plexus	60 Gy preferred, 66 Gy maximum
OAR pharynx	Mean dose <50 Gy
Parotid gland	Mean dose to at least 1 gland 26 Gy OR at least 20 cc of the combined volume of both parotid glands to <20 Gy OR at least 50% of 1 gland to <30 Gy
Submandibular gland	Mean dose <39 Gy
Glottic larynx	Mean dose <45 Gy—lower if possible
Cervical Esophagus	Reduce as much as possible (<30 Gy)
Lips	Mean dose <20 Gy; maximum dose <35 Gy (<50 Gy for oral cavity lesions)
Oral cavity minus PTV	Mean dose <30 Gy (uninvolved)
Mandible, tempero-mandibular joint	70 Gy preferred; no more than 1 cc, >75 Gy
Eyes	Maximum dose <50 Gy
Cochlea	No more than 5% >55 Gy
Lens	Maximum dose <8–10 Gy
Unspecified tissue (outside targets)	No more than 5% can receive > prescription dose; no more than 1% or 1 cc of unspecified tissue can receive 110% of the prescription dose

*When base of skull (BOS) involvement, the BOS constraints can be used from RTOG 0615. Protocols state that all PTV regions are subtracted from OAR structures when assessing DVHs.
Note: DVH parameters can be exceeded if needed to ensure adequate tumor coverage.

■ Alternative techniques to avoid the need to feather the junction include the following:
- ■ Dynamic field matching technique: involves continuously moving the superior border of the AP field from 1.5 cm below the central axis

(ie, match line) to 1.5 cm above the central axis, creating in effect a 3 cm match line (2). No field junctions are necessary.

- "Gradient matching" technique: involves modifying the superior border of the AP field so that the total dose per fraction (eg, 2 Gy) is delivered in three separate segments, with only about one-third of the dose delivered at the superior-most aspect of the original field. This creates a broad dose gradient along the match line (no field junctions necessary). One must be careful to extend the IMRT target 1 to 2 cm into the AP field to ensure that the inverse planning system accounts for this deliberate "underdosing" and ensures adequate coverage (3).

- Replanning
  - Patient/tumor geometry frequently changes during the course of treatment because of tumor and normal tissue shrinkage and/or weight loss of the patient. As such, some advocate for replanning during the course of therapy, particularly for IMRT, in which dosimetric goals may be significantly compromised for small anatomic changes given the steep dose gradients.
  - Some have found significant overdosing of critical structures without replanning (4); others have found replanning to be limited to parotid sparing only (5).
  - Both the need to replan and the ideal frequency of replanning remain an area of controversy and active investigation.

OROPHARYNX CANCER

Site-Specific Indications

- Radiotherapy (+/- chemotherapy) is indicated for an organ preservation treatment approach.

Target Volumes

- GTV/PTV: as per general principles
- CTV: include levels II through IV and retropharyngeal/parapharyngeal nodes. Include level Ib if BOT, tonsil, or level II and III nodes are involved. Level V is included for any N+ or tonsil/BOT primary and may be excluded for T1-2, N+ (6).

Radiotherapy

Special Considerations

- For well-lateralized T1-2/N0-1 tonsil tumors, consider unilateral irradiation, including primary tumor + ipsilateral levels II–IV only. Can use IMRT, mixed electron-photon beam (4:1) with open neck technique (tumors <5 cm deep), or wedged pair in supine position (tumors >5 cm deep; Figure 4.4).

▪ For pharyngeal wall tumor, inferior border is extended more than 3 cm beyond the pharyngeal wall mass to include the entire pharynx in initial fields; the posterior border for the tumor boost/cone down is placed immediately anterior to the spinal cord. Daily verification images are required.

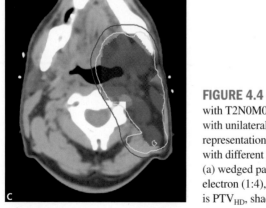

FIGURE 4.4 A 53-year-old man with T2N0M0 SCC of L tonsil treated with unilateral irradiation. Axial representations of dose distributions with different planning techniques: (a) wedged pair, (b) mixed photon-electron (1:4), (c) IMRT. Shaded red is PTV$_{HD}$, shaded blue is PTV$_{ED}$.

LARYNX CANCER

Site-Specific Indications

■ Conventional radiotherapy alone is the standard treatment for early-stage glottic cancer. Concurrent chemoradiotherapy is indicated for laryngeal preservation in locally advanced disease. For patients with extensive bone/cartilage involvement, total laryngectomy + postoperative (chemo)radiotherapy is preferred.

Target Volumes

■ Early-stage glottic cancer (T1N0 or T2N0)
  ■ For early-stage glottic tumor, no elective nodal irradiation is required. Field is generally 5 × 5 or 6 × 6 cm with opposed laterals (Figure 4.5a and b). Consider unilateral field for disease involving 1 cord (Figure 4.5c).
■ Borders are as follows:
  ■ Superior: top of thyroid cartilage for T1, additional 1 cm higher for T2.
  ■ Anterior: flash anteriorly
  ■ Posterior: anterior margin of vertebral bodies. Can cone down with this border moved anteriorly by 0.5 to1 cm to spare arytenoids and avoid late laryngeal edema. This can be done *only* in the absence of gross disease in the posterior half of the vocal cords (Figure 4.5d).
  ■ Inferior: lower edge of cricoid cartilage for T1, as low as possible without treating through the shoulders for T2
■ IMRT is not recommended in this setting.
■ Consider nodal irradiation for extensive supraglottic/subglottic extension as risk of occult nodal metastases is higher.
■ All other stages of larynx cancer
  ■ GTV/PTV: as per general principles
  ■ CTV: include levels II through IV. Include level V for any N+ or extension to the BOT. Include retropharyngeal nodes if extension to pharyngeal wall (possibly glossopharyngeal sulcus) or BOT.

Special Considerations

■ For early-stage glottic cancer (T1N0), hypofractionation has improved local control compared with standard fractionation. Recommended dose is 63 Gy/2.25 Gy/fx or 66 Gy/2.2 Gy/fx.
■ For T2N0 glottic cancer, especially lesions with impaired vocal cord mobility, consider treating to 65.25 Gy/2.25 Gy/fx or to 74.4 Gy/1.2 Gy/fx twice daily, or accelerated concomitant boost technique, or treating with 6 fx weekly. Some advocate the addition of radiosensitizing chemotherapy in this setting.

FIGURE 4.5 A 53-year-old man with T1N0 SCC of the L true vocal cord for definitive radiation. (a) DRR of lateral field. (b) Axial representations of dose distribution with opposed laterals with wedges. (c) Axial representation of dose distribution with unilateral field only. (d) Sagittal demonstration of lateral field with optional cone down to reduce dose to arytenoids.

◼ After total laryngectomy, include tracheal stoma if subglottic extension, emergency tracheostomy through tumor, soft tissue of neck invasion, +ECE, +tracheal margin, or surgical scar crossing the stoma.

HYPOPHARYNX CANCER

Site-Specific Indications

◼ Concurrent chemoradiotherapy is indicated for organ preservation in advanced disease. For patients with extensive bone/cartilage involvement, total laryngopharyngectomy + postoperative (chemo)radiotherapy is preferred.

Target Volumes

- GTV/PTV: as per general principles
- CTV
  - CTV_{HD} = GTV + 5 mm
  - CTV_{ED} includes bilateral levels Ib to V, and retropharyngeal/parapharyngeal nodes for all cases.

Special Considerations

- Care must be taken not to underestimate the inferior extent of the disease (toward the apex) because it is very difficult to appreciate on endoscopic exam or on imaging. If matching laterals/IMRT to AP field, match below the cricoids, or as low as necessary, to achieve margin on disease (do not match over tumor). Coverage of superior esophagus may be necessary.

NASOPHARYNX CANCER

Site-Specific Indications

- Definitive chemoradiotherapy is standard for nasopharyngeal cancer. Exception is T1N0 when recommendation is radiation alone.

Target Volumes

- GTV/PTV: as per general principles. MRI fusion can delineate intracranial OARs, locate tumor infiltration, and visualize nerves that need to be included.
  - CTV_{HD} = GTV + 5 mm
  - CTV_{ED} (per RTOG 0615) = the entire nasopharynx, anterior one-half to two-thirds of the clivus (entire clivus, if involved), skull base (foramen ovale and rotundum bilaterally must be included for all cases), pterygoid fossae, parapharyngeal space, inferior sphenoid sinus (in T3–T4 disease, the entire sphenoid sinus), and posterior fourth to third of the nasal cavity and maxillary sinuses (to ensure pterygopalatine fossae coverage). The cavernous sinus should be included in high-risk patients (T3, T4, bulky disease involving the roof of the nasopharynx). Include bilateral levels Ib to V and retropharyngeal/parapharyngeal nodes for all cases.

Special Considerations

- Level Ib nodes may be spared in N0 patients, or N+ only in retropharyngeal or level IV nodes.
- If hard palate, nasal cavity, or maxillary antrum is involved, bilateral IB nodes must be covered.

■ CTV$_{HD}$ margin can be reduced to 1 mm for tumors in close proximity to critical structures (eg, tumor invading clivus and abutting, but not involving, brainstem). However, CTV$_{HD}$ margin should not be reduced if disease is frankly invading the critical structure.

MAJOR SALIVARY GLAND CANCER

Site-Specific Indications

■ Radiotherapy is generally indicated in the postoperative setting and for locally advanced disease (T3/4, N+) or T1/2, N0 with high-risk features (high grade, + margin, PNI, LVSI, adenoid cystic histology) or recurrent disease.
■ When surgery is not feasible, neutron therapy has shown some advantage.

Target Volumes (Postoperative)

■ CTV (parotid)
  ■ For low-grade, N0 tumors: parotid bed only.
  ■ For high-grade, N0 tumors (nonadenoid cystic histology): consider electively treating levels Ib, II, III.
  ■ For N+ tumors: parotid bed + ipsilateral levels I–V.
  ■ For all cases with extensive facial nerve invasion, or adenoid cystic histology, cover facial nerve pathway up to the base of the skull. Focal PNI is not an indication.
■ CTV (submandibular)
  ■ Aside from small, low-grade tumors with N0 neck, cover ipsilateral levels I to IV electively, even in N0 neck. Cover level V if N+. If named nerve is extensively involved (eg, lingual, hypoglossal), cover up to base of skull.
■ PTV: as per general principles

Special Considerations

■ Set up patient with "open-neck" technique to expose ipsilateral neck; consider bolus to ensure adequate superficial coverage over surgical bed.
■ IMRT planning is favored for improved homogeneity and reduced dose to contralateral critical structures. Other planning techniques include a wedge pair or mixed photon/electron fields (Figure 4.4).

ORAL CAVITY CANCER

Site-Specific Indications

■ Radiotherapy for oral cavity cancers is indicated for use in the postoperative setting for T3/4, pN2/3, close/positive margins, PNI, LVSI, deep muscle invasion, and +ECE.

Target Volumes (Postoperative)

■ CTV: postoperative bed + draining lymphatics include ipsilateral levels Ia/b, II, and III when electively treating. If high-risk disease, or N+, treat ipsilateral levels I to V. Consider contralateral neck irradiation if primary lesion approaches midline (eg, floor of mouth and central mobile tongue).

■ PTV: as per general principles

Special Considerations

■ When treating lip (eg, with electrons) or buccal mucosa lesion, consider inserting a lead block (with wax on either side to prevent backscatter) to shield gingiva/teeth/tongue.

■ For large (T3) or high-grade T2 upper lip lesions, treat facial lymphatics electively with a moustache field (see image in subsection on nasal cavity).

■ For medically inoperable patients, consider a combination of external beam RT (40–50 Gy) + brachytherapy or intraoral cone boost (20–25 Gy).

CANCER OF UNKNOWN PRIMARY

Site-Specific Indications

■ Radiotherapy is used for carcinoma of unknown primaries of the H&N region, after neck dissection as primary treatment.

Target Volumes

■ CTV: in general, include pharyngeal axis (include base of skull and post one-third of the nasal cavity to ensure margin on the nasopharynx) and bilateral levels Ib to V as well as retropharyngeal nodes, with the following exceptions:

■ Squamous cell carcinoma (SCC) found in unilateral-level Ib node only: treat bilateral levels I to V.

■ SCC found in one parotid LN may be related to primary skin cancer of the scalp: treat ipsilateral levels II to V, parotid, and preauricular nodes. Take skin cancer history and examine scalp for primary lesion.

■ For adenocarcinoma histology metastatic to parotid, parotidectomy is required and helps guide field design.

■ For p16+ disease, cover oropharynx +/- nasopharynx; do not cover hypopharynx/larynx

■ If p16 status unavailable, but unilateral level II LN only, consider sparing hypopharynx/larynx

■ PTV: as per general principles

Special Considerations

- For patients with a single node without ECE, observation after a neck dissection is recommended.
- Isolated SCV metastases are usually from a primary below the clavicles; comprehensive pharyngeal axis irradiation is usually not offered.
- For adenocarcinoma histology, parotidectomy is required and helps guide field design.
- If matching fields via monoisocentric technique, place isocenter as low as possible above the shoulders.

MAXILLARY SINUS CANCER

Site-Specific Indications

- Radiotherapy is indicated in the postoperative setting for all but small, low-grade tumors that have been completely resected with adequate margins.

Target Volumes

- CTV (postoperative)
    - MRI fusion is recommended to help delineate intracranial organs at risk and areas of tumor infiltration and also helps visualize nerves that need to be included.
    - Carefully review operative report for extent of disease spread, paying attention to invasion of pterygopalatine fossa, orbital wall, cribiform plate, and cranial nerve foramina.
    - CTV includes the tumor bed + 5 to 10 mm margin.
    - Consider a boost to high-risk areas (+margin, PNI) in this volume.
- PTV: as per general principles. IGRT is preferred to limit margins and help reduce dose to critical structures (ie, optic nerves).

Special Considerations

- Fill all air cavities or surgical defects with obturator or water-filled balloon to improve dose homogeneity.
- IMRT planning is preferred given high doses in proximity to critical structures (eg, optic apparatus; Figure 4.6a and b).
- If orbit is uninvolved, treat up to the medial limbus of the eye (exclude lens and retina). If involved, treat the entire eye while trying to shield the lacrimal gland if uninvolved by disease.
- Elective nodal irradiation is controversial in this setting. For N+ disease, treat bilateral IB-V if the patient can tolerate treatment.

FIGURE 4.6 A 66-year-old woman with T4N0M0 SCC of the R maxillary sinus, s/p endoscopic resection for postoperative radiotherapy to tumor bed only (nodal regions not electively treated). (a) Axial, (b) sagittal, and (c) coronal images displaying isodose distributions. Shaded blue is PTV. (d) DVH of treatment plan.

NASAL CAVITY/VESTIBULE CANCER

Specific Indications

■ Radiotherapy is indicated for smaller lesions (may be cosmetically superior to surgery) or postoperatively for locally advanced lesions.

Target Volumes

■ GTV/PTV (definitive): per general principles
■ CTV (nasal vestibule)
  ■ For tumors <2 cm or well-differentiated tumors, treat GTV + 2 cm margin.
  ■ For tumors ≥2 cm or poorly differentiated tumors, treat GTV + 2 cm margin + bilateral facial lymphatics ("moustache field") and levels Ib to II bilaterally (Figure 4.7a and b).
  ■ For N+ disease, treat levels I to V bilaterally.
■ CTV (nasal cavity)
  ■ Treat GTV + 2 cm margin.
  ■ LN not treated electively if confined to nasal cavity.
  ■ Tumors that involve superior nasal cavity are often treated with similar field arrangement to maxillary sinus tumors.

Special Considerations

■ Fill nasal cavity with wax to reduce dose heterogeneity.
■ Interstitial brachytherapy can be used for nasal septum lesions.
■ Cartilage invasion is not a contraindication to definite radiotherapy.

THYROID CANCER

Indications

■ External beam radiotherapy is generally used postoperatively for well-differentiated follicular/papillary cancer in the setting of pT4 and age ≥45 years, gross residual disease after I-131, and lesions with inadequate radioactive iodine uptake with +margin, or +ECE; for all resected anaplastic carcinoma; or for medullary carcinoma that is either locally advanced or associated with an elevated calcitonin level postoperation without evidence of distant disease.

Target Volumes

■ CTV (postoperative)
  ■ Include surgical bed, cervical/SCV/mediastinal nodes at risk.

FIGURE 4.7 An 83-year-old woman treated with definitive radiation for T1N1M0 neuroendocrine carcinoma of the left nasal cavity. Representative (a–c) axial and (d) coronal images are displayed. Shaded red is GTV, thick green line is CTV, and thick blue line is PTV. Note inclusion of facial lymphatics encompassing the region included in traditional "moustache field."

- If superior mediastinal nodes are involved, cover entire mediastinum (to subcarinal region). If not, can electively treat superior mediastinum only.
- PTV: per general principles (Figure 4.8a and b)

FIGURE 4.8 A 27-year-old woman with multiple recurrent papillary thyroid cancer, s/p thyroidectomy and reresection for local recurrence with bilateral lymph node dissection with ECE receiving postoperative radiation 63 Gy / 30 fx (2.1 Gy/fx). Representative (a) axial and (b) coronal CT slices showing PTV1 and PTV2 with (c) DVH. Note inclusion of upper mediastinal lymphatics.

Special Considerations

- Reduce dose to oropharynx and oral cavity as much as possible.
- For 3D CRT, often treatment is AP/posteroanterior initially (42–44 Gy for cord tolerance), then boost tumor bed + ipsilateral neck only with opposed (off-cord) obliques.

NONMELANOMATOUS HEAD AND NECK SKIN CANCER

Indications

■ Radiotherapy is used in the definitive setting (ie, around nose, ear, and eyelids) for cosmetically superior results, or in the postoperative setting for high-risk or recurrent tumors.

Target Volumes

■ GTV (definitive): done clinically
■ CTV (definitive)
  ■ Generally, GTV + 1 cm margins (2 cm for large infiltrative tumors)
  ■ May reduce margin around critical structures (eg, eye and lip).
  ■ Nodal areas are treated for large, poorly differentiated SCC, or parotid LN +, or N2/3 disease.
■ CTV face/neck (postoperative): tumor bed + ipsilateral neck nodes + parotid gland (if not removed) + involved named nerves (trigeminal, facial) up to base of skull.
■ CTV scalp (postoperative): cover tumor bed + 2 cm margin or in large infiltrative/recurrent tumors, treat whole scalp. IMRT can be used.
■ PTV: per general principles

Special Considerations

■ Radiation is delivered with either orthovoltage X-rays (75–125 kVp) or electrons (6–12 MeV). Use skin bolus for electrons. Orthovoltage has a maximum dose at the surface, and less beam constriction at depth. Electrons have sharper dose fall off and are more widely available.
■ Use eye shield for eyelid lesions.
■ Doses (definitive): >2 Gy dose per fraction is preferred. Frequently used doses include the following: 60 Gy/2.5 Gy/fx, 55 Gy/2.75 Gy/fx, 45 Gy/3 Gy/fx, or 66 to 70 Gy/2 Gy/fx for large tumor abutting critical structures (eg, eye). Doses of 40 Gy/4 Gy/fx, 30 Gy/6 Gy/fx, or 20 Gy/10 Gy/fx are effective regimens when cosmesis is less of a priority.
■ Dose (postoperative): standard fractionation 60 Gy to tumor bed and 54 Gy to operative bed and elective nodes. Boost areas of +margin, ECE, PNI.

HEAD AND NECK MELANOMA

Indications

■ Radiotherapy is used primarily in the postoperative setting for tumor thickness >4 mm with ulceration or satellite lesions, +margin, N+, or recurrent disease. Desmoplastic histology is controversial.

Target Volumes

- CTV (postoperative): tumor bed + ipsilateral nodal levels II to IV
- PTV: per general principles

Special Considerations

- Because of the relatively radioresistant histology, higher dose per fraction has been advocated. In the postoperative setting, acceptable regimens include 48 to 50 Gy/2.4 to 2.5 Gy/fx and 60 to 66 Gy/2 to 2.2 Gy/fx for +margins, +ECE.
- In primary/palliative setting, 30 Gy/6 Gy/fx twice weekly and 50 Gy/2.5Gy/fx are commonly accepted regimens.
- For melanoma of the scalp, planning options include mixed photon/electron technique versus IMRT versus brachytherapy (7).
- Can consider "sandwiching" bolus material between 2 thermoplastic masks to ensure consistent setup.

REFERENCES

1. Ahn PH, Garg MK. Positron emission tomography/computed tomography for target delineation in head and neck cancers. *Semin Nucl Med.* 2008;38:141–148.

2. Duan J, Shen S, Spencer SA, et al. A dynamic supraclavicular field-matching technique for head-and-neck cancer patients treated with IMRT. *Int J Radiat Oncol Biol Phys.* 2004;60:959–972.

3. Amdur RJ, Liu C, Li J, et al. Matching intensity-modulated radiation therapy to an anterior low neck field. *Int J Radiat Oncol Biol Phys.* 2007;69:S46–S48.

4. Hansen EK, Bucci MK, Quivey JM, et al. Repeat CT imaging and replanning during the course of IMRT for head-and-neck cancer. *Int J Radiat Oncol Biol Phys.* 2006;64:355–362.

5. Wu Q, Chi Y, Chen PY, et al. Adaptive replanning strategies accounting for shrinkage in head and neck IMRT. *Int J Radiat Oncol Biol Phys.* 2009;75:924–932.

6. Sanguineti G, Califano J, Stafford E, et al. Defining the risk of involvement for each neck nodal level in patients with early T-stage node-positive oropharyngeal carcinoma. *Int J Radiat Oncol Biol Phys.* 2009;74:1356–1364.

7. Wojcicka JB, Lasher DE, McAfee SS, et al. Dosimetric comparison of three different treatment techniques in extensive scalp lesion irradiation. *Radiother Oncol.* 2009;91:255–260.

5 Breast Radiotherapy

Steven C. Oh and Rahul D. Tendulkar

GENERAL PRINCIPLES

- Radiation therapy for patients with breast cancer can range from treatment of a tumor bed to chest wall and comprehensive regional nodal radiation fields.
- Patient and disease factors guide the choice of treatment technique.
- Common principles are used when planning radiation therapy, in the setting of both limited and radical surgery.

Localization, Immobilization, and Simulation

- Localization: spiral CT with 3 mm slices spanning the neck to the upper abdomen
- Immobilization: patient is positioned supine or prone (for patients with large or pendulous breast).
  - Cradles, indexed angled breast boards, and prone immobilization devices may be customized to optimize treatment planning.
  - Positioning for external beam radiation is adjusted to limit skin contact at the inframammary sulcus.

- Treatment through the contralateral breast may be avoided by displacing and immobilizing the contralateral breast and by prone positioning techniques.
- Footrests and knee supports help keep patients from sliding down boards. Attaching the breast board to the treatment table makes the immobilization system more rigid, translating into more reproducible treatments.
- Simulation: radiopaque wires are used to delineate target volumes and on all surgical scars.

Target Volumes and Organs of Interest Definition

- Breast: all breast tissue defined clinically and by imaging
- Lumpectomy cavity
  - Included for all patients treated with partial mastectomy

FIGURE 5.1 Lymph node groups displayed on digitally reconstructed AP radiograph (a) and axial image at the level of the proximal clavicle (b). Green indicates level I; blue, level II; yellow, level III; red, SCV lymph nodes.

- Cavity includes seroma and may be determined with the combination of physical examination, computed tomography (CT), ultrasound, and identification of surgical clips (1).
- Chest wall is delineated by landmarks used for external beam breast conservation therapy.
- Lymphatics
  - Axillary nodal groups are referenced to the pectoralis minor muscle— the level I nodes are lateral, level II are deep, and level III are medial to pectoralis minor (Figure 5.1).
  - SCV lymph node groups are referenced to the axillary vein.
  - Internal mammary (IM) chain fields include the IM nodes at the first 3 intercostal spaces.

Treatment Planning

- CT–based 3D planning is favored over 2D planning to reduce normal tissue dose and better delineate target areas.
- Segmented planning and intensity-modulate radiotherapy (IMRT) may improve dose homogeneity and conformality, respectively.

Critical Structures

- Heart: especially relevant to treatment of left-sided breast cancer and IM fields
  - 40 Gy to less than the whole organ
- Lung: especially relevant for SCV fields matched to low breast or chest wall tangent fields
  - V20 to 20%

Technical Factors

- 6 MV photons used for separation <23 cm; higher-energy photons may be needed for larger separations
  - Use of higher energy beams may underdose superficial tissues
- Dose homogeneity may be improved by use of higher-energy photons and with tissue compensators, including physical wedges, dynamic wedges, segmented field technique (2), and IMRT (3).
- Tumor bed boost fields typically use an en face electron beam.
  - Electron energy selected so that 80% or 90% isodose line (IDL) covers tumor bed (CTV) with a 2 cm expansion
- Dose distribution is calculated with heterogeneity correction
- Optimize plans to result in no more than 5% to 8% dose variation, with maximum dose not exceeding 15% of the prescription

■ Special cases: respiratory gating and/or deep-inspiration breath-holding techniques may be required to reduce normal tissue doses.

WHOLE BREAST RADIOTHERAPY

Introduction

■ Breast conservation techniques include whole-breast and partial-breast radiation.
■ Combinations of multiple photon fields and electron fields are used.

Localization, Immobilization, and Simulation

■ Immobilization: patient is positioned supine on angled breast board (typically 10° to 15°) with the ipsilateral hand positioned above the head; the head is rotated toward the contralateral breast.
  ■ Board is angled to make the chest wall parallel to the table, to decrease the amount of collimation used.
  ■ To avoid bolus effect, additional immobilization may be used to limit skin contact at the inframammary sulcus (eg, custom mesh bra or mold).
  ■ Avoiding treatment through the contralateral breast may be accomplished by rotating the gantry and/or displacing and immobilizing the contralateral breast.
■ Simulation: radiopaque wires are placed to delineate tangent fields and on all surgical scars (Figure 5.2).
  ■ Isocenter is placed at least D_{max} depth from surface and typically in a central or deeper location.

FIGURE 5.2 Simulation—arm above the head with radiopaque wires (arrows) delineating the target region and scar.

Breast Conservation—External Target Volumes and Organs of Interest Definition

■ CTV = residual breast tissue and lumpectomy cavity

Treatment Planning

■ Tangent fields
- ■ Field borders: field borders are delineated with radiopaque wires taped to the skin as follows:
  - Superior: 1 cm above the breast tissue (usually at the inferior aspect of the clavicle or the sternal manubrium joint)
  - Inferior: 2 cm below the inframammary line
  - Medial: mid-sternum
  - Lateral: mid-axillary line
  - Position of the field borders should be modified based on the location of the lumpectomy cavity and areas at higher risk of recurrence.
- ■ Medial and lateral tangents: encompass all breast, with posterior edge of beam through medial and lateral radiopaque wires.
  - Rotate the gantry to achieve a flat border posteriorly
  - Rotate the collimator to decrease the amount of lung in field to 3 cm or less (typically 2 cm), with flash of 2 cm anteriorly (Figure 5.3a).
  - High tangent field with border typically at the level of the humeral head may be considered when electing for additional axillary coverage (Figure 5.3b).
  - Table rotation or a block may be placed at the superior aspect of the tangent fields to reduce divergence into a matched SCV field.
  - Caution when using a heart block for patients with inferiorly located tumors, as underdosing of the tumor bed may occur (4).
- ■ Dose homogeneity may be improved with tissue compensators (eg, physical or dynamic wedges).
  - Avoid medial physical wedges due to concern for scatter radiation dose to the contralateral breast.
  - Segmented field technique may reduce hotspots receiving high dose.
    - Forward planning is used to create multiple segments of varying field size, blocking portions of the field that are contributing to the high-dose area.
    - IMRT can accomplish a similar effect.
■ Boost field
- ■ The lumpectomy cavity is delineated on planning CT. Ultrasound may aid in delineating the lumpectomy cavity, particularly when the breast tissue is dense and the seroma and/or tumor bed is small (5).

FIGURE 5.3 Standard breast tangent field (a), and "high" breast tangent field (b). Green indicates level I; blue, level II; yellow, level III; red, SCV lymph nodes. Boost field (c) (15 MeV electrons, 100 SSD).

- En–face field encompassing the scar and lumpectomy cavity with a 2 cm margin.
- An electron energy encompassing the lumpectomy cavity with the 80% to 90% isodose line is chosen (typically 9–16 MV electrons; Figure 5.3c).

Dose/Fractionation

- Conventionally fractionated radiotherapy for whole breast is 45 to 50.4 Gy/1.8 to 2 Gy/fx over approximately 5 weeks.
- Hypofractionated schedules include 40 to 42.5 Gy/2.66 Gy/fx daily and 39 Gy/3 Gy/fx every other day (6,7).
  - Typically limited to patients with medial-lateral separation of 25 cm or less (6)
- Boost dose is typically 10 to 16 Gy/2 Gy/fx.

LYMPH NODE (LN) RADIOTHERAPY

Introduction

- SCV and IM lymph node radiation is given for patients at higher risk of regional recurrence.
- The primary technical consideration with lymph node treatment planning is field matching to breast and chest wall tangent fields.

Localization, Immobilization, and Simulation

- Patient is set up and immobilized as described in the "General Principles" section.
- To match an SCV photon field to breast tangents, two techniques may be considered for the tangent fields:
  - Multiple isocenter technique
    - Breast tangent fields are set up as described in the "Breast Conservation—External Beam Radiotherapy" section.
    - For each tangent, the table is rotated away from the gantry to eliminate superior divergence.
    - A corner block must be placed in the superior aspect of the tangent field to avoid overlap of the collimated tangent field
  - Single isocenter technique (monoisocentric)
    - Isocenter is placed at the match line, which is the superior aspect of the tangent field.
    - A half-beam block is used to eliminate superior divergence.
    - Multileaf collimators are used to define a 2 to 3 cm lung bite
    - This technique is limited by field size and the inability to rotate the collimator on the tangent fields.

Target Volumes and Organs of Interest Definition

- Use the subclavian vessels and intercostal spaces as reference (8). IV contrast may help delineate nodal regions.
- SCV fields include the high axillary (levels II and III), infraclavicular, and SCV lymph nodes.
- IM lymph node borders
  - Encompass the first 3 intercostal spaces
  - Medial border is the ipsilateral sternal edge or 1 cm medial to the IM vessels if the distance to the sternum is more than 1 cm.
  - The volume extends laterally to include the IM vessels with a 5 mm margin, posteriorly to the pleura and anteriorly to the anterior extent of the IM vessels (9).

Treatment Planning

- SCV field (Figure 5.4a)
  - Superior: inferior cricoid cartilage, ensuring that skin is not flashed.
  - Inferior: inferior aspect of the clavicular head (this is the level of the isocenter). Placement above the inferior aspect of the clavicular head may result in underdosing of the level III lymph nodes by the SCV field (10).
  - Medial: at vertebral pedicles.
  - Lateral: If specifically targeting the axillary lymph nodes, then place the lateral border lateral to the humeral head; conversely, the lateral border could be placed at the medial aspect of the humeral head if not specifically targeting axillary lymph nodes. The acromioclavicular joint is usually blocked superolaterally.
  - Angle the SCV field 10° to 15° off cord by rotating the gantry.
  - Use a half-beam block inferiorly.
  - Prescription was historically to a depth of 3 cm; however, with CT planning, prescribing to the delineated target volumes ensures adequate dose (11).
- Axillary boost field (Figure 5.4b)
  - PA field may be used to supplement dose to the mid-axillary plane for patients at high risk of axillary failure.
  - Simulated in the same fashion as an AP SCV field; however, lung blocking is used, and the superior-medial border is moved to the edge of the clavicle.
  - Alternatively, IMRT may be considered (12).
- IM Fields (Figure 5.4c–f)
  - IM lymph nodes can be treated by expanding the tangent fields or by matching a separate medial electron field to shallow tangent fields (13). Choice of technique depends on the patient's anatomy and is driven by risk of normal tissue toxicity (9).
  - "Wide" or "deep" tangents include IM nodes by moving the medial border toward the contralateral breast; however, at increased lung dose.
  - Partially wide tangents treat the IM nodes and block the heart from the photon field (Figure 5.4c and e). An electron field may supplement dose to the chest wall blocked in the partially wide tangents.
  - An electron field matched to photon tangents is angled to account for the bowing of the isodose distribution (Figure 5.4d and f); the electron field width should be at least 4 cm to allow for adequate dose buildup. A matched photon or mixed photon/electron field (typically 20:80 or 30:70 ratio) may also be considered.

FIGURE 5.4 SCV radiation field (a); posterior axillary boost (b); deep tangent field (c) (IM LN are delineated in red), matched electron IM LN field (d); projection of partially wide tangents (e); and electron field matched to tangents fields (f) used to treat IM LN on a woman after mastectomy. The matched electron field may be separated into multiple fields of different energies to spare deep structures such as heart and lung.

Dose/Fractionation

- SCV field: 45 to 50 Gy/1.8 to 2 Gy/fx daily
- Axillary boost field is given simultaneously to bring mid-axillary dose typically to 45 Gy.
- IM field: 45 to 50 Gy/1.8 to 2 Gy/fx daily

PRONE BREAST RADIOTHERAPY

Introduction

- Prone breast techniques aid in delivering radiation therapy to patients with large or pendulous breasts.
- Advantages of prone positioning include the following:
  - Movement of target tissue away from the chest wall
  - Reduced skin folds
  - Reduced lung or heart volume in the radiation field
- Disadvantages of prone positioning include the following:
  - Heart displacement anteriorly (a particular disadvantage for tumor beds near the chest wall)
  - Interference of positioning devices with portal imaging
  - Difficulty visualizing the light fields
  - Uncomfortable patient positioning
  - Inability to treat regional LN

Localization, Immobilization, and Simulation

- The patient is set up prone on a specially designed immobilization device with arms above the head, allowing for the ipsilateral breast to be displaced from the chest wall (Figure 5.5a and b).
- The contralateral breast is displaced laterally so as not to interfere with the tangent fields (Figure 5.5c).
- Ipsilateral breast is marked with radiopaque wires as described for supine techniques. Tangential fields are designed as in supine techniques; however, they typically include less lung (often referred to as "lung bite"; Figure 5.5d). Relative to a supine technique, chest wall and breast movement in the prone position is minimal.
- If tumor bed is not accessible for en–face boost, repeat simulation in the supine position may be necessary.

Target Volumes and Organs of Interest Definition

- As with supine positioning, fields target breast tissue and lumpectomy CTV.
- As opposed to supine techniques, less lung is typically included in the field. As a result, portions of the chest wall may typically receive less dose.

FIGURE 5.5 Prone positioning device (a); patient with cancer of the left breast positioned prone to allow breast tissue to fall anteriorly (b); contralateral breast displaced posteriorly (c); typical treatment port (d); and isodose distribution achieved (e) for a patient for whom dose was prescribed to the 98% IDL using 6 MV photons, field-within-field technique, no wedges.

The degree of chest wall included in the treatment field can be adjusted based on the location of the tumor.

Treatment Planning

- Treatment planning principles for prone positioning are the same as those used in supine positioning.
- The main dosimetric advantage is a decreased skin fold at the inframammary sulcus and decreased separation from entrance to exit.
- Chest wall and lung receive less dose than would be expected in a supine position (Figure 5.5e).

Dose/Fractionation

■ Dose and fractionation for prone positioning are the same as those used in supine positioning.

ACCELERATED PARTIAL BREAST RADIOTHERAPY

Introduction

■ Balloon catheter brachytherapy, multicatheter interstitial brachytherapy, intraoperative techniques, and 3D conformal RT (3DCRT) using photon or electron fields are the predominant treatment techniques.
■ Only balloon catheter brachytherapy technique will be discussed here, based on the NSABP B-39/RTOG 0413 protocol.

Simulation

■ Balloon is placed in lumpectomy cavity at the time of surgery or postoperatively under ultrasound guidance.
■ Balloon is filled with saline (30–70 mL) mixed with 1 to 2 mL contrast.
■ Patient is positioned supine with the ipsilateral hand positioned above the head; the head is rotated toward the contralateral breast.
■ CT images from mandible to several centimeters below the inframammary sulcus (inclusive of entire lung) are produced.

Target Volumes and Organs of Interest Definition

■ PTV: 10 mm circumferential expansion around the balloon, less the balloon volume. Regions 5 mm from the skin surface and area of the chest wall/pectoralis muscles are excluded from PTV.
■ Air and fluid trapped around the balloon are delineated.

Treatment Planning

■ Tissue–balloon conformance: %PTV coverage ([vol trapped air/vol PTV] × 100) should equal 90% or higher. Adequate PTV coverage cannot be achieved if this value is less than 90% and the percentage of PTV displaced is greater than 10%. Ninety percent or greater of the prescribed dose should cover 90% or greater of the PTV.
■ Balloon symmetry: balloon geometry should be within 2 mm of expected dimensions.
■ Minimal balloon surface–skin distance: 7 mm or greater is optimal; however, 5 to 7 mm is acceptable. Skin dose maximum is 145% or lower of prescription dose (Figure 5.6).

FIGURE 5.6 Woman with a brachytherapy balloon catheter in place; 50% to 150% isodose lines from ^{192}Ir source are displayed.

- Normal tissue dose volume parameters: volume of tissue receiving 150% (V150) and 200% (V200) of the prescribed dose is limited to 50 cc or lower and 10 cc or lower, respectively.
- Uninvolved normal breast: less than 60% of the whole-breast volume should receive 50% or greater of the prescribed dose. Balloon volume is subtracted from the breast volume.

Dose/Fractionation

- Brachytherapy: high-dose rate (HDR): 34 Gy/10fx prescribed at 1 cm from the balloon surface. Treatments are delivered BID over 5 to 7 days with an interfraction interval of 6 hours or more.
- 3DCRT: 38.5 Gy/3.85 Gy/fx delivered BID over 5 to 7 days with an interfraction interval of 6 hours or more.

POSTMASTECTOMY RADIOTHERAPY

Introduction

- Postmastectomy radiotherapy includes chest wall treatments and may extend to target nodal regions.
- Combinations of photon and electron fields may be used to individualize treatments.
- Techniques include standard tangents (± matched IM node fields), electron fields, wide tangents, and partially wide tangent fields. A "reverse hockey stick" technique involves AP/PA photon fields treating the SCV lymph nodes and lateral chest wall matched to a medial electron field targeting the

medial chest wall and IM lymph nodes (this will not be discussed in this section).

■ Immediate breast reconstruction is discouraged when postmastectomy radiotherapy is part of an overall treatment plan (14). A delayed or two-stage reconstruction may be preferred. Challenges with breast reconstructions include:

    ■ Coverage of IM lymph nodes may be compromised

    ■ Tangent angle selection can be impacted

    ■ Flexibility of electron-only chest wall treatment is eliminated

Localization, Immobilization, and Simulation

■ The patient is set up in a supine position on a breast board and CT scan is conducted as described in the "General Principles" section.

■ Contralateral breast tissue or measurements made prior to radical surgery may be used to delineate the superior, inferior, medial, and lateral field dimensions (particularly for patients with inflammatory breast cancer and those who have undergone bilateral mastectomy).

■ Similar landmarks to those used in breast conservation are delineated with radiopaque wire taped to the skin (inferior aspect of clavicular head, mid-sternum, mid-axillary line, 2 cm below the level of the contralateral infra-mammary sulcus).

■ Photon tangents (Figure 5.7a)

    ■ Medial and lateral tangents are designed with posterior edge of beam through medial and lateral radiopaque wires.

    ■ Blocking and table rotation are used to reduce divergence into a matched SCV field.

    ■ The medial border may be moved toward the contralateral breast/chest wall to provide additional coverage of IM lymph nodes (ie, wide or partially wide tangents, see "Lymph Node Radiotherapy" section).

    ■ Isocenter is placed at least D_{max} from the skin surface for photon tangent fields.

■ Electron fields (Figure 5.7b)

    ■ After delineation of the chest wall target volume, the field is broken into multiple en face fields (typically 2 fields).

    ■ Isocenter for each field located at the skin surface.

■ Boost field: en–face electrons encompassing the scar with 3 to 5 cm margin, using energy sufficient for the 90% IDL to encompass the surface-to-chest-wall thickness (Figure 5.7c).

■ Description of matching nodal fields is described in the "Lymph Node Radiotherapy" section.

FIGURE 5.7 Isodose distribution from tangent photon fields (a) and matched electron fields (b). Mixed 6 and 10 MV photons with 25° wedges prescribed to the 96% isodose line using 5 mm tissue equivalent bolus were used for the photon fields. A medial field of 9 MV electrons and a lateral field of 12 MV electrons, 100 SSD at skin surface using 5 mm tissue equivalent bolus were used for the electron fields. An en–face boost with a 3 cm radial margin on the mastectomy scar was designed for an electron boost (c).

Target Volumes and Organs of Interest Definition

■ CTV = the entire chest wall (skin surface to rib–soft tissue interface)
   ■ IM nodes are typically included although not specifically targeted unless disease factors warrant doing so.
   ■ Ipsilateral SCV volumes should be delineated if they are to be targeted.
■ A scar boost may be considered if there is high risk of local recurrence (eg, positive or close margins and inflammatory breast cancer).
■ Lung and heart volumes are delineated.

Treatment Planning

- Tissue-equivalent bolus material may be applied at the time of simulation or modeled with virtual simulation.
- For inflammatory breast cancer patients and others, bolus may be applied at the beginning of treatment and titrated to effect with the goal of brisk erythema at the completion of therapy.
  - Bolus at 3 to 10 mm can be utilized on a daily or every-other-day schedule, with regular assessment of skin erythema.
  - Clinical judgment must be used when determining duration of bolus use.
- Dose heterogeneity corrections should be applied unless artifact because metal components in tissue expanders are present.
- Photon tangents
  - Treatments are typically prescribed to the 95% isodose line.
  - Optimized dose homogeneity may require tissue compensators (eg, physical wedges, dynamic wedges, and IMRT).
  - Standard tangents typically have less coverage of IM nodes; however, a lower V20 is usually achieved.
  - Partially wide tangents to treat the IM nodes may help reduce dose to the heart.
- Electron fields
  - Overlapping fields, also known as "hot matching," may be done to ensure adequate coverage of junctions; however, a noticeable match-line fibrosis may result.
  - Junction shifts of 0.5 cm every 5 fractions may be used to reduce the risk for match-line fibrosis.
  - Electron energy is selected such that the 90% IDL encompasses the chest wall thickness to the anterior pleural surface (typically 6–12 MV electrons); this would also serve as the prescription isodose line.

Dose/Fractionation

- Chest wall and nodal fields receive 45 to 50.4/1.8 to 2 Gy/fx daily.
- Boost field delivers 10 to 16 Gy/2 Gy/fx.
- Inflammatory breast cancer: consider 1.5 Gy per fx BID (≥6-hour interfraction interval) to 51 Gy delivered to the chest wall and regional nodes, followed by a 15 Gy boost to the chest wall with electrons. Brisk erythema at the completion of treatment is desirable.
- The mid-axilla may be supplemented in high-risk cases (see "Lymph Node Radiotherapy").

REFERENCES

1. Goldberg H, Prosnitz RG, Olson JA, et al. Definition of postlumpectomy tumor bed for radiotherapy boost field planning: CT versus surgical clips. *Int J Radiat Oncol Biol Phys.* 2005;63:209–213.

2. Ludwig V, Schwab F, Guckenberger M, et al. Comparison of wedge versus segmented techniques in whole breast irradiation: effects on dose exposure outside the treatment volume. *Strahlenther Onkol.* 2008;184:307–312.

3. Descovich M, Fowble B, Bevan A, et al. Comparison between hybrid direct aperture optimized intensity-modulated radiotherapy and forward planning intensity-modulated radiotherapy for whole breast irradiation. *Int J Radiat Oncol Biol Phys.* 2009;76:91–99.

4. Raj KA, Evans ES, Prosnitz RG, et al. Is there an increased risk of local recurrence under the heart block in patients with left-sided breast cancer? *Cancer J.* 2006;12:309–317.

5. Berrang TS, Truong PT, Popescu C, et al. 3D ultrasound can contribute to planning CT to define the target for partial breast radiotherapy. *Int J Radiat Oncol Biol Phys.* 2009;73:375–383.

6. Whelan T, MacKenzie R, Julian J, et al. Randomized trial of breast irradiation schedules after lumpectomy for women with lymph node–negative breast cancer. *J Natl Cancer Inst.* 2002;94:1143–1150.

7. Bentzen SM, Agrawal RK, Aird EG, et al. The UK Standardisation of Breast Radiotherapy (START) Trial A of radiotherapy hypofractionation for treatment of early breast cancer: a randomised trial. *Lancet Oncol.* 2008;9:331–341.

8. Madu CN, Quint DJ, Normolle DP, et al. Definition of the supraclavicular and infraclavicular nodes: implications for three-dimensional CT-based conformal radiation therapy. *Radiology.* 2001;221:333–339.

9. Pierce LJ, Butler JB, Martel MK, et al. Postmastectomy radiotherapy of the chest wall: dosimetric comparison of common techniques. *Int J Radiat Oncol Biol Phys.* 2002;52:1220–1230.

10. Garg AK, Frija EK, Sun TL, et al. Effects of variable placement of superior tangential/supraclavicular match line on dosimetric coverage of level III axilla/axillary apex in patients treated with breast and supraclavicular radiotherapy. *Int J Radiat Oncol Biol Phys.* 2009;73:370–374.

11. Liengsawangwong R, Yu TK, Sun TL, et al. Treatment optimization using computed tomography–delineated targets should be used for supra-clavicular irradiation for breast cancer. *Int J Radiat Oncol Biol Phys.* 2007;69:711–715.

12. Wang X, Yu TK, Salehpour M, et al. Breast cancer regional radiation fields for supraclavicular and axillary lymph node treatment: is a posterior axillary boost field technique optimal? *Int J Radiat Oncol Biol Phys*. 2009;74:86–91.

13. Arthur DW, Arnfield MR, Warwicke LA, et al. Internal mammary node coverage: an investigation of presently accepted techniques. *Int J Radiat Oncol Biol Phys*. 2000;48:139–146.

14. Motwani SB, Strom EA, Schechter NR, et al. The impact of immediate breast reconstruction on the technical delivery of postmastectomy radiotherapy. *Int J Radiat Oncol Biol Phys*. 2006;66:76–82.

6   Thoracic Radiotherapy

Jason W. D. Hearn and Gregory M. M. Videtic

GENERAL PRINCIPLES

- General principles for planning thoracic radiotherapy (TRT) are valid across a range of malignancies and include simulation techniques, definition of dose-limiting structures, dose constraints, and beam setups.
- Specific dose prescriptions are determined by tumor types and treatment approaches, whether preoperative, definitive, or postoperative therapy.

Localization, Immobilization, and Simulation

- Volumetric treatment planning: computed tomography (CT) simulation on a flat surface for definition of gross tumor volume (GTV)
- Patient position: supine with arms raised above head
- Immobilization:
  - Numerous systems (eg, vacuum-lock bag and thermoplastic mold) are commercially available to position the arms above the head in a reproducible, patient-friendly manner.

- Pancoast tumor may require arms akimbo.
- Localization: contiguous spiral CT slices with 3 mm slice acquisition from the level of the cricoid cartilage to the lowest ribs, including the liver.
- Contrast agents: as indicated clinically.
  - Oral contrast to delineate esophagus.
  - Intravenous contrast to delineate major blood vessels.
- Treatment planning FDG-PET/CT scan done with the patient in treatment position is desirable.
  - Otherwise, staging positron emission tomography (PET) done prior to simulation may be coregistered with simulation CT for contouring, mindful of positional and table differences.
- Target
- Motion due to respiration must be identified and accounted for as indicated. There is a range of valid approaches (see Chapter 2 for details):
  - Four-dimensional CT
  - Physical control/restriction of tumor motion
  - Gating/fiducials
  - Free breathing

Target Volumes and Organs of Interest

- Reference should be made to the 1993 International Commission on Radiation Units & Measurements report (ICRU)-62 document for a complete description of the various target volume definitions (GTV, CTV, and PTV).
- Normal anatomy to be routinely identified
  - Lungs: right and left done separately, then combined as a composite lung volume.
  - Heart: from its base (RTOG definition: beginning at the CT slice where the ascending aorta originates and encompassing the great vessels) to the apex
  - Esophagus: from the bottom of the cricoid to the gastroesophageal junction
  - Spinal cord: should be contoured on each CT slice.
  - Brachial plexus, stomach, liver, kidneys, and other structures: as needed based on the clinical scenario and tumor location.

Treatment Planning

- 3D conformal therapy (3DCRT): published outcomes largely based on TRT planning, with combinations of coplanar or noncoplanar 3D conformal fields, without heterogeneity corrections or accounting for tumor motion.
- Intensity-modulated radiation therapy (IMRT): Increasingly being used in the chest. In the setting of IMRT, clinicians must be able to control respiratory motion to limit excursion.

- The National Cancer Institute "Guidelines for the Use of IMRT" can be found on the following website: www.qarc.org/Protocols/IMRTGuidelines.pdf.
- Normal tissue constraints are prioritized when planning in the following order:
  - Spinal cord: highest priority dose constraint, irrespective of other constraints
    - Must not exceed 50.5 Gy to any contiguous volume ≥0.03 cc
  - Lung: the percentage of *total* lung volume that receives >20 Gy (the V20) should not exceed 37%. Alternatively, the mean lung dose should optimally be <20 Gy
    - Total lung volume = combined lungs minus the CTV
  - Esophagus: mean dose is optimally <34 Gy but is not an absolute requirement. V55 <33% is also another reference value.
    - Heart (proportions are of the whole organ)
      - 60 Gy to <1/3
      - 45 Gy to <2/3
      - 40 Gy to <3/3
      - mean dose <30 Gy is increasingly recommended.
  - Brachial plexus ≤66 Gy

Technical Factors

Beam energies
- Photon energies: 6 to 10 MV; higher energy photons (>10 MV) are not recommended in lung tissue as the beam penumbra increases and the beam edge becomes less sharp. Also, the periphery of the tumor may be underdosed (due to the greater build-up region), especially with small field sizes.

Beam shaping
- Multileaf collimation or individually shaped (5 HVL) custom blocks for normal tissue protection.

Heterogeneity Corrections

- Historically, TRT plans used "uncorrected" dose calculations that replace all body tissue by a water equivalent, ie, homogeneous dose deposition-assuming homogenous tissue electron densities.
- Currently, TRT distinguishes the heterogeneous nature of tissues in the chest to more appropriately predict dose deposition, normal tissue toxicities, and outcomes. Therefore, heterogeneity corrections are now recommended in general treatment planning (see Chapter 1 for more details).

Image-guided radiotherapy (IGRT)

■ Multiple forms of IGRT are commercially available, some of which include cone beam CT, CT-on-rails, orthogonal radiographs, infrared tracking, and fiducial-based systems.

■ Use of image guidance improves reliability of treatment setup and delivery and, thus, in some scenarios, may permit reduction of daily set-up margins.

Proton beam therapy (PBRT)

■ Use of PBRT for TRT is an active area of investigation for its potential impact on normal tissue toxicities.

■ Use of PBRT in TRT delivery has been challenging due to the large impact of motion on proton dosimetry.

NON-SMALL CELL LUNG CANCER

TRT Indications

■ Definitive TRT with concurrent chemotherapy is the standard of care for patients with stage III unresectable non-small cell lung cancer (NSCLC) and selected inoperable stage II patients.

■ Preoperative or postoperative TRT may be indicated in selected stage II or III NSCLC patients.

Target Volume Definitions

A. Definitive TRT (see Figure 6.1)

■ GTV = primary tumor + clinically positive nodes seen on planning CT (>1 cm short axis diameter) or pretreatment PET (SUV >3) and any histologically proven involved nodal level (by mediastinoscopy, endobronchial ultrasound-guided biopsy, etc.)
  ■ Contour primary tumor using "lung windows" setting.
  ■ The volumes may be disjointed or noncontinuous.
■ In the event of a collapsed lobe/lung segment, PET may be helpful to distinguish tumor from fluid/atelectasic lung.
■ CTV = GTV + 0.5 to 1 cm margin to account for microscopic extension.
  ■ If an ITV is used, CTV = ITV + 0.5 to 1 cm.
  ■ Elective nodal irradiation (ENI)
    • Until recently, standard TRT practice in the United States has been to deliver dose electively to nonclinically involved hilar, mediastinal, and/or supraclavicular nodal areas.

FIGURE 6.1 (a, b) Axial and (c, d) coronal images of a 50-year-old male with T2aN3M0, stage IIIB CLC of the left lower lobe with bilateral supraclavicular (SCV) involvement treated to 60 Gy in 30 fractions with concurrent chemotherapy. CTV is shown in red with PTV in green.

- Modern imaging techniques (especially PET) and studies of nodal failure patterns have shifted practice away from ENI to include only grossly involved or high-risk nodal basins in the target.
- Remains an area of investigation.
- PTV (will reflect approaches to motion management and any IGRT use)
- Breath-hold or gating (non-ITV) approach
  - PTV margin = CTV +1 cm in the superior/inferior direction and 0.5 cm in the axial plane, with daily imaging
- ITV approach
  - PTV = CTV + 0.5 to 1 cm. If daily IGRT used, margins reduced to 0.5 cm.
  - For free-breathing, non-ITV approach
  - PTV = CTV + 1.5 cm superior/inferior and at least 1 cm in axial plane.

B. Preoperative RT (Figure 6.2a and b)

- GTV, CTV, PTV: per definitions used in section A above
- Consider
  - Inclusion of nodal stations adjacent to involved nodes
  - Nodal stations connecting involved stations if skip metastases present

C. Postoperative TRT (Figure 6.2c and d)

- Reference preoperative imaging (CT and PET), operative note, pathology report, and any additional staging procedures/biopsies if applicable

FIGURE 6.2 (a) Axial and (b) coronal images of a 45-year-old female with left Pancoast tumor, T3N0M0, stage IIB, treated with neoadjuvant chemoradiation (45 Gy/25 fx with concurrent cisplatin and etoposide) followed by resection and adjuvant chemotherapy (CTV shown in red). (c) Axial and (d) coronal images of a 59-year-old female with T3N0M0 NSCLC of the right upper lobe, stage IIB, s/p resection with a questionable chest wall margin treated with adjuvant radiation (50 Gy/25 fx) and chemotherapy (sequential; CTV shown in red).

- CTV should include, at a minimum:
  - Bronchial stump
  - Ipsilateral hilum
  - Pathologically involved nodal stations
  - Consider
    - Inclusion of nodal stations adjacent to involved nodes
  - Nodal stations connecting involved stations if skip metastases are present
    - Any nodal stations connecting involved stations when skip metastases are present.
  - CTV for positive margins/extracapsular extension should reference:
  - Preoperative GTVs
    - Surgical clips
    - Operative reports
    - Pathology report

Treatment Planning

Dose/Fractionation

- A. Definitive TRT: 60/2 Gy/fx
  - Figure 6.3 is a representative dose-volume histogram (DVH) for definitive TRT
- B. Preoperative RT: 45 to 50.4 Gy at 1.8 to 2 Gy/fx followed by surgery at 4 to 6 weeks
- C. Postoperative TRT:
  - R0 resection: 45 to 50 Gy
  - R1 resection: 54 to 60 Gy
  - R2 resection: 60 to 66 Gy for gross/residual disease
  - 2 Gy fraction size recommended

SMALL CELL LUNG CANCER

TRT Indications

- "Early start" TRT (with cycles 1 or 2 of chemotherapy (1,2)) is recommended for definitive treatment of limited stage disease.

Target Volume Definitions

- GTV = primary tumor and involved nodes (PET positive or >1 cm in diameter on CT)

FIGURE 6.3 Dose-volume histogram for definitive chemoradiation in a 65-year-old female with stage IIIA NSCLC treated with 60 Gy/30 fx via 4-field technique.

- CTV = GTV + 1.5 to 2 cm margin
  - Elective nodal irradiation (see NSCLC for review).
    - Elective nodal irradiation remains controversial but is generally not recommended.
- PTV = 0.5 to 1 cm expansion of CTV, depending on tumor motion management
- Special considerations
  - Pre-TRT chemotherapy can influence target delineation.
  - In patients with radiographic complete response after chemotherapy, ipsilateral hilum/mediastinum should be treated.
  - When TRT is delivered after chemotherapy initiation, the use of prechemotherapy target volumes as opposed to postchemotherapy volumes has been studied, with postchemotherapy volumes preferred for the primary tumor delineation (3).

Dose/Fractionation

- 45 Gy/1.5 Gy/fx with twice-daily fractions, interfraction interval ≥6 hours (4)
- Alternative schedules:
  - 40 Gy at 2.67 Gy/fx over three weeks (2)
  - 70 Gy/ 2 Gy/fx from nonrandomized studies

THYMOMA

TRT Indications

- TRT for thymoma is most commonly used in the adjuvant setting. Adjuvant TRT routinely indicated for resected thymic carcinomas.
- Definitive TRT (+/- chemotherapy) for medically inoperable or surgically unresectable patients

Target Volume Definitions

- Fuse available preoperative imaging to TRT planning CT images for target definition.
- GTV = there is generally no gross disease after resection; note placement of surgical clips in relation to the preoperative tumor.
- CTV = surgical bed/resected volume; generally no nodal targets
- PTV = CTV + 1 cm; target motion minimal

Treatment Planning

- Classical field arrangements for resected thymoma include: "wedged pair" (Figure 6.4) or anteroposterior/posteroanterior fields (AP/PA) with anterior weighting.

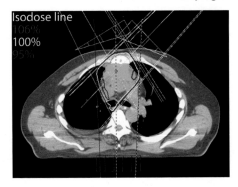

FIGURE 6.4 Axial planning CT image from a 56-year-old male with resected Masaoka stage II thymoma, WHO type C; postoperative TRT, 60 Gy/2 Gy/fx, 3-field plan (incorporating a wedged pair), mixed 6 MV and 10 MV photons.

Dose/Fractionation

- R0 resection: 45 to 50 Gy
- R1 resection: 54 to 60 Gy
- R2 resection: 60 to 66 Gy for gross/residual disease
- 2 Gy fraction size recommended

ESOPHAGEAL CARCINOMA

TRT Indications

- The role of TRT in the definitive management of esophageal cancer is controversial.
- Preoperative, definitive, and postoperative TRT are all advocated, depending on institutional and clinician preference.
- Cervical esophageal carcinomas have historically been judged unresectable and treated with definitive TRT +/- chemotherapy.

Special Considerations at Simulation

- For cervical and upper-third thoracic lesions, immobilization with a mask is preferred.
- Oral contrast and intravenous contrast may improve visualization of the esophageal mass or strictures to help with contouring. In the postoperative setting, oral contrast is not given.
- There is currently no defined role for motion compensating techniques.

Target Volume Definitions

Definitive TRT (see Figure 6.5a)

- GTV = gross tumor and PET-positive regional lymph nodes
- CTV = GTV + 4 cm proximally and distally and + 1 cm radially
- PTV = CTV + 1 to 2 cm proximally and distally and + 1 cm radially
- Preoperative/postoperative TRT
- Essentially replicates definitive fields.
  - In postoperative setting, fields may need to be modified for + margin.
- Use CT and PET imaging to define primary and nodal target contours (Figure 6.5b and c).

FIGURE 6.5 Axial (a) and sagittal (b) representative CT images from a 72-year-old male with adenocarcinoma of the distal esophagus, T3N1M0, stage IIIA, treated with definitive chemoradiation (50.4 Gy/28 fx). CTV is shown in red and PTV in green. (c) Axial and (d) sagittal images from a 55-year-old male with adenocarcinoma of the distal esophagus, T3N2M0, stage IIIB, treated with adjuvant radiation (50.4 Gy/28 fx) with concurrent chemotherapy. CTV is shown in red.

Dose/Fractionation

- Definitive TRT: 50.4 Gy/1.8 Gy/fx
  - The use of brachytherapy boost in the definitive setting is controversial (5).
- Preoperative TRT: dose ranges from 41.4 to 50.4 Gy/1.8 to 2 Gy/fx.
- Postoperative radiation dose: 45 to 50.4 Gy/1.8 to 2 Gy/fx (6,7).

MESOTHELIOMA

TRT Indications

- Definitive TRT is indicated adjuvantly after extrapleural pneumonectomy (EPP)
- Prophylactic RT to drain/biopsy sites (now very controversial)
- Palliative TRT for pain from uncontrolled disease progression

Special Considerations at Simulation

- Visualize incision/drainage sites with radiopaque material.
- Consider bolus on the chest wall to ensure adequate dose delivery to the scar or any drain sites, with a 2 to 4 cm margin.

Target Volume Definitions (Figure 6.6a–c)

- Surgical clips aid in the delineation of medial preresected diaphragm, inferior diaphragmatic insertion, and sternopericardial recess.
- GTV = generally not applicable
- CTV = all ipsilateral pleural surfaces, including the chest wall from the apex to the lung bases, pericardium, diaphragmatic crural insertions, any surgical mesh reconstruction, ipsilateral hilum, and mediastinal boundary, with inclusion of all surgical clips
  - Particular attention is to be paid to identifying and contouring the posterior and inferior aspects of the insertions of the diaphragm.
- Boost volumes
  - Ipsilateral mediastinum in the setting of resected N2 disease
  - Positive margins/gross residual disease PTV = CTV + 5 to 8 mm expansion

Dose/Fractionation

- R0 resection: 54 Gy/2 Gy/fx to ipsilateral hemithorax
- R1 resection: 60 Gy/2 Gy

FIGURE 6.6 Treatment planning images for a 70-year-old man with a pT2N0M0 malignant mesothelioma post EPP; adjuvant TRT, 54 Gy/2 Gy/fx; IMRT, 10 MV photons. Axial (a), coronal (b), and sagittal (c) images are shown, with PTV depicted in blue. Note the costophrenic angles and sternopericardial recess.

Planning Considerations (see DVH; Figure 6.7)

- IMRT is recommended in the setting of adjuvant TRT (Table 6.1; 8,9).
  - Mean lung dose of intact lung <10 Gy.

STEREOTACTIC BODY RADIOTHERAPY FOR LUNG TUMORS

Indications

- Medically inoperable T1/T2N0M0 NSCLC
- Oligometastatic disease to the lungs in selected patients

Special Considerations at Simulation

- Rigid immobilization
- Tumor range of motion to be kept to less than 1 cm (methods as detailed in "General Principles, Target Motion").

FIGURE 6.7 Dose-volume histogram for the IMRT plan of the patient receiving 54 Gy after EPP depicted in Figure 6.6.

Target Volume Definitions

■ GTV = lung lesion, as drawn on "lung windows" setting of free-breathing CT scan
■ CTV = GTV
■ ITV = target representing the range of GTV motion through the breathing cycle (see Figure 6.8)

TABLE 6.1 IMRT Recommendations for Post-EPP TRT (10)

Target or Organ	Dose Goal or Constraint
PTV (CTV + 5–7 mm)	>95% coverage with 54 Gy
Intact lung	<20% to receive >20 Gy; <60% to receive >5 Gy; mean dose, <10 Gy
Liver	<30% to receive >30 Gy
Kidney	<20% to receive >15 Gy
Heart	<50% to receive >45 Gy
Spinal cord	<10% to receive >45 Gy; no portion to receive >50 Gy
Esophagus	<30% to receive >55 Gy; mean dose <34 Gy

FIGURE 6.8 A 57-year-old man with medically inoperable NSCLC of the right upper lobe, treated on an SBRT protocol: 30 Gy/1 fx. (a) From the CT simulation, this image depicts the GTV during free breathing (red), at maximum inhalation (green), and maximum exhalation (blue). (b) ITV (lime) was generated by combining GTVs. PTV (light blue) = ITV + 5 mm. Isodose distribution using a 6-arc plan, 6 MV photons, prescribed to the 80% isodose line (c).

- PTV = ITV + 3 to 10 mm margin; expansion will reflect the parameters of the particular delivery system, tumor motion control approach, and dose planning algorithm for a given institution

Treatment Planning

- North American collaborative group standard set by RTOG 0236 protocol
- May include 3D, IMRT, helical-based approaches, CyberKnife®.

- General goals of planning
  - Delineation of all normal thoracic structures
  - All organs at risk to have detailed dose constraints, defined both by maximum point dose and by volume
  - Dose constraints vary by fractionation schedules.
  - Coverage of at least 95% of the PTV by prescription isodose curve, with tight control of dose spillage around the target

Dose/Fractionation

- RTOG 0236 schedule: 60 Gy/20 Gy/fx with an interfraction interval >40 hours and <7 days over 8 to 14 days; other regimens frequently used: 48 Gy/12 Gy/fx and 50 Gy/10 Gy/fx

REFERENCES

1. Jeremic B, Shibamoto Y, Acimovic L, et al. Initial versus delayed accelerated hyperfractionated radiation therapy and concurrent chemotherapy in limited small-cell lung cancer: a randomized study. *J Clin Oncol.* 1997;15:893–900.

2. Murray N, Coy P, Pater JL, et al. Importance of timing for thoracic irradiation in the combined modality treatment of limited-stage small-cell lung cancer. The National Cancer Institute of Canada Clinical Trials Group. *J Clin Oncol.* 1993;11:336–344.

3. Kies MS, Mira JG, Crowley JJ, et al. Multimodal therapy for limited small-cell lung cancer: a randomized study of induction combination chemotherapy with or without thoracic radiation in complete responders; and with wide-field versus reduced-field radiation in partial responders: a Southwest Oncology Group Study. *J Clin Oncol.* 1987;5:592–600.

4. Turrisi AT, III, Kim K, Blum R, et al. Twice-daily compared with once-daily thoracic radiotherapy in limited small-cell lung cancer treated concurrently with cisplatin and etoposide. *N Engl J Med.* 1999;340:265–271.

5. Gaspar LE, Winter K, Kocha WI, et al. A phase I/II study of external beam radiation, brachytherapy, and concurrent chemotherapy for patients with localized carcinoma of the esophagus (Radiation Therapy Oncology Group Study 9207): final report. *Cancer.* 2000;88:988–995.

6. Macdonald JS, Smalley SR, Benedetti J, et al. Chemoradiotherapy after surgery compared with surgery alone for adenocarcinoma of the stomach or gastroesophageal junction. *N Engl J Med.* 2001;345:725–730.

7. Bedard EL, Inculet RI, Malthaner RA, et al. The role of surgery and postoperative chemoradiation therapy in patients with lymph node positive esophageal carcinoma. *Cancer.* 2001;91:2423–2430.

8. Forster KM, Smythe WR, Starkschall G, et al. Intensity-modulated radiotherapy following extrapleural pneumonectomy for the treatment of malignant mesothelioma: clinical implementation. *Int J Radiat Oncol Biol Phys.* 2003;55:606–616.

9. Ahamad A, Stevens CW, Smythe WR, et al. Intensity-modulated radiation therapy: a novel approach to the management of malignant pleural mesothelioma. *Int J Radiat Oncol Biol Phys.* 2003;55:768–775.

10. Miles EF, Larrier NA, Kelsey CR, et al. Intensity-modulated radiotherapy for resected mesothelioma: the Duke experience. *Int J Radiat Oncol Biol Phys.* 2008;71:1143–1150.

7 Gastrointestinal (Nonesophageal) Radiotherapy

Monica E. Shukla, Kevin L. Stephans,
and May Abdel-Wahab

GENERAL PRINCIPLES

- General principles relevant to EBRT planning of gastrointestinal (GI) malignancies include simulation techniques, definition of dose-limiting structures, dose constraints, and planning principles.
- Specific dose prescription will be determined by tumor types and treatment approaches, for example, preoperative, definitive, or postoperative therapy.

Localization, Immobilization, and Simulation

- Volumetric treatment planning (CT simulation on a flat surface) for the definition of gross tumor volume (GTV), clinical target volume (CTV), and planning target volume (PTV).
- Patient position: specific to tumor site and stage.

- Immobilization: arms raised above the head. A range of immobilization systems are available. The use of a "belly board" for small bowel displacement may be appropriate for a range of GI malignancies.
- Contiguous spiral computed tomography (CT) slices acquired with 3 to 5 mm slice acquisition
  - For pancreas and stomach tumors, obtain images from above the diaphragm to below the kidneys.
  - For rectal and anal cancers, obtain images from the L3 vertebral body to 6 in. below an external anal marker.
- Contrast agents and fiducial/tumor markers
  - Oral contrast is used to delineate the small bowel. One should allow a 2-hour transit time for the agent through the small bowel.
  - Intravenous (IV) contrast to delineate the tumor and lymph nodes (LN); alternatively, may fuse contrasted diagnostic CT scan to the planning images.
  - Barium enema may help delineate rectal and anal tumors.
    - This will influence the use of heterogeneity corrections in treatment planning and may displace the tumor.
    - If contrast is used, a scan without contrast should also be obtained to define a lesion's "natural" position and to aid with heterogeneity collections.
  - For rectal and anal malignancies, a marker at the level of the anus aids the determination of the inferior field borders.
  - In postsurgical patients, the location of surgical clips matched to preoperative imaging can aid in the delineation of the resected tumor bed.
    - NB: surgery alters normal anatomy, so clips should be used for reference only.
    - Clip placement may not reflect tumor location, for example, hemostasis clip versus tumor resection margin.

Target Volumes and Organs of Interest Definition

- Reference should be made to the 1993 International Commission on Radiation Units & Measurements (ICRU) report 62 document for complete description of various target volume definitions (GTV, CTV, and PTV).
- Normal anatomy to be routinely identified for pancreas/gastric cancer
  - Liver
  - Small bowel
  - Kidneys
  - Spinal cord
- Normal anatomy to be routinely identified for rectal/anal cancer
  - Small bowel
  - Bladder
  - Femoral heads: to be contoured inferiorly to the level of ischial tuberosity

- External genitalia
- Consider remaining large bowel
- Consider iliac crest when using intensity-modulated radiation therapy

Treatment Planning

Therapy

- Two-dimensional, anatomy-based planning has been the historic standard, from which the majority of data on treatment results and toxicity outcomes have conventionally been derived. Elective nodal irradiation of non-clinically involved regional lymphatics was standard in this approach.
- 3-Dimensional conformal radiotherapy (3DCRT) contemporary treatment paradigms for GI malignancies use planning based on CT-derived targets, for which combinations of coplanar 3D conformal fields are used for external beam radiotherapy (EBRT) delivery.
- Intensity-modulated radiation therapy (IMRT): IMRT is increasingly used in radiotherapy (RT) treatment of the GI tract. Its main advantage lies in potential reduction in normal tissue toxicity.

Critical Structures

- Spinal cord: maximum dose, less than 50 Gy.
- Liver: two-thirds of the organ, less than 48 Gy; mean dose, less than 32 Gy (in normal liver function).
- Kidneys: a renal perfusion scintiscan may be obtained prior to treatment to assess kidney function.
  - The equivalent of one whole kidney should be limited to less than 20 Gy.
  - The mean dose for the total kidneys is less than 16 Gy.
  - If the patient has only one functioning kidney, exclude two-thirds of that kidney from the radiation field.
- Small bowel: maximum point dose, less than 54 Gy; 1 cc, less than 50 Gy; 20 cc, less than 45 Gy. Relative volume limits: up to 10% may receive 54 Gy; up to 15%, 50 Gy.
- Stomach: maximum dose, 54 Gy. Relative volume limits: up to 10% may receive 54 Gy; up to 15%, 50 Gy.
- Femoral head: maximum dose, 50 Gy.
- Iliac crests: No more than 5% above 50 Gy; no more than 50% above 30 Gy (Radiation Therapy Oncology Group [RTOG] 0529) (1).
- External genitalia: No more than 5% above 40 Gy, no more than 50% above 20 Gy (RTOG 0529).
- Bladder: No more than 5% above 50 Gy; no more than 50% above 35 Gy (RTOG 0529) (1).

Technical Factors

■ 6 to 18 MV photon beam energies; higher-energy photons are often required for patients with greater separation.

■ Beam shaping with multileaf collimators or individually shaped (5 HVL) custom blocks for normal tissue protection outside the target volume.

■ Heterogeneity corrections: if using contrast-enhanced CT scans at the time of planning, density overrides or fusion of noncontrasted scans are required when using heterogeneity corrections in planning.

■ Avoid planning on CT images with contrast enemas if near tumor because of displacement effects.

PANCREATIC CANCER

Indications

■ Postoperative (adjuvant) chemoradiotherapy

■ Definitive chemoradiotherapy for unresectable (T4) disease

■ Preoperative (neoadjuvant) chemoradiotherapy in selected patients

■ Chemoradiotherapy with 5FU

Localization, Immobilization, and Simulation

■ Immobilization and patient position
  ■ Supine.
  ■ Can consider prone with belly board in patients who will not have AP/PA field contributions.

■ Contrast agents and markers
  ■ Oral contrast to delineate the small bowel.
  ■ IV contrast to delineate the tumor and LN. Specific use of pancreatic contrast timing protocols will improve resolution.

Target Volume Definition

Neoadjuvant

■ GTV
  ■ Primary tumor + clinically positive LN greater than 1 cm short axis diameter
    • Involved volume best defined on contrast-enhanced magnetic resonance imaging (MRI) or pancreatic phase contrast-enhanced CT scan.

- CTV
  - May elect to include immediate primary LN drainage, with a focus only on the highest-risk portions of these chains for neoadjuvant therapy.
    - Head lesions: consider celiac, porta hepatis, suprapancreatic and pancreatic duodenal LNs.
    - Tail lesions: consider celiac, splenic, and lateral suprapancreatic LNs.
- PTV
  - PTV = CTV + 1 cm.

Adjuvant
- GTV
  - None. If STR, then treat remaining GTV per unresectable and include LN below.
- CTV
  - Tumor bed plus nodal drainage for initial field with a boost to the tumor bed.
    - Tumor bed defined by fusion of preoperative imaging and surgical clips.
- Pancreaticojejunostomy and hepaticojejunostomy (if the entire jejunum is resected, do not include pancreaticogastrostomy).
  - At-risk LN
    - Head lesions: celiac (proximal 1 to 1.5 cm of the celiac artery), superior mesenteric (proximal 2.5 cm of the superior mesenteric artery), porta hepatis, suprapancreatic, pancreaticoduodenal, para-aortic (from T11 to L3).
    - Tail lesions: celiac, superior mesenteric, splenic, lateral suprapancreatic.
    - Coverage of the porta hepatis and pancreaticoduodenal lymph nodes should be attempted for body/tail lesions but may be omitted to meet dose constraints on the kidneys.
- PTV
  - PTV = CTV + 1 cm

Unresectable
- GTV
  - Primary tumor + clinically positive LN greater than 1 cm short axis diameter.
    - Involved volume best defined on contrast-enhanced MRI or pancreatic phase contrast-enhanced CT scan.

■ CTV
- ■ Historically, primary draining LN, as listed in the "Adjuvant" section, were included in the CTV; current practice trends are to restrict the size of the CTV to GTV plus 1 cm, then a margin for PTV margin, given limited ability to control primary disease.
■ PTV
- ■ PTV = CTV + 1 cm

Treatment Planning

■ 4-field technique
- ■ Initial AP/PA fields:
  - • Superior border: T10/T11 vertebral body interspace.
  - • Inferior border: L3/L4 vertebral body interspace.
  - • Lateral borders: 2 to 3 cm on preoperative primary tumor extent or gross tumor, no less than 2 cm from the vertebral bodies.
- ■ Initial lateral fields
  - • Superior/inferior borders: same as AP/PA fields.
  - • Anterior border: 1.5 to 2 cm anterior to anterior aspect of preoperative primary tumor or gross tumor and at least 3.5 to 4 cm anterior to the anterior edges of the vertebral bodies.
  - • Posterior border: split the vertebral bodies in half.
- ■ Boost field: 1.5 to 2 cm margin on gross tumor or preoperative primary tumor extent.
  - • Beam arrangement: while AP/PA and 3-field plans incorporating AP/PA and laterals +/- wedges are most common, oblique fields (particularly moving the lateral beams toward anterior obliques) may reduce kidney doses, and noncoplanar beam arrangements may reduce small bowel doses (Figures 7.1 and 7.2).

Volumetric Planning Goals

- ■ 95% of the PTV should receive at least 95% of the prescription dose.
- ■ No portion of the PTV should receive less than 90% of the prescription dose.
- ■ 99% of the CTV should receive at least 95% of the prescription dose.
- ■ 0.1 cc of tissue is limited to 115% of the prescription dose.
- ■ 1.0 cc of tissue (or 5% of PTV) is limited to 110% of the prescription dose.
- ■ 5 cc of tissue (or 10% of PTV) is ideally limited to 105% of the prescription dose.

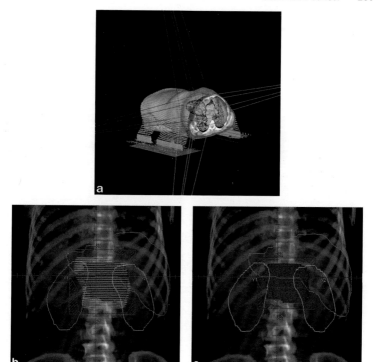

FIGURE 7.1 A 72-year-old woman with borderline resectable pancreatic adenocarcinoma involving the portal vein was treated with neoadjuvant chemoradiation. EBRT technique: 4-field noncoplanar beam arrangement optimized liver sparing (a). The initial fields (b) covered the primary tumor (red) and immediate primary LN drainage (green) with 1 cm radial and 1.5 cm superior/inferior block margins. The cone down (c) covered the primary tumor with 1 cm block margins.

Dose/Fractionation

- Conventional fractionation: 1.8 Gy/fx
- Neoadjuvant RT: 45 Gy to CTV, boost GTV to 50.4 to 54 Gy
- Adjuvant RT: 45 Gy to CTV, boost tumor bed and pathologically involved LN regions to 50.4 Gy
- Definitive RT: 50.4 to 54 Gy to GTV

FIGURE 7.2 A 51-year-old man, post-Whipple procedure for adenocarcinoma of the pancreatic head. EBRT plan: 4-field noncoplanar beam arrangement optimized liver sparing (a). The initial fields (b) covered the tumor bed (red) and associated LN (green). The cone down (c) covered the tumor bed with a 2 cm block margin. The tumor bed was delineated by fusion of the preoperative CT scan (d) to the planning CT scan (e).

GASTRIC CANCER

Indications

■ Postoperative chemoradiotherapy is the most typical indication, with rare selected cases of preoperative chemoradiotherapy or definitive chemoradiotherapy for unresectable disease.

Localization, Immobilization, and Simulation

■ Immobilization and patient position
  ■ Supine with arms above the head.
■ Contrast agents and markers
  ■ Oral contrast to delineate the small bowel.
  ■ IV contrast to delineate the tumor and LN.

Target Volume Definition

Adjuvant

■ GTV
  ■ If STR, then treat remaining GTV per unresectable and include LN as below.
■ CTV
  ■ Tumor bed
    • Coverage of tumor bed elective for resected T1 to T2a lesions with wide margins.
    • Include for all stage T2b to T4.
    • Defined by fusion of preoperative imaging and surgical clips.
    • Preoperative endoscopy reports may help determine surgical bed location.
  ■ Remaining stomach (include 5 cm of normal esophagus for gastroesophageal junction [GEJ] lesions)
    ■ If perigastric or other nodal involvement.
    ■ If surgical margins less than 5 cm.
  ■ Lymph nodes
    • If nodal involvement (LN) or T4 disease, LN at risk defined by the location of the primary tumor.
      • GEJ: perigastric, periesophageal, and celiac.
      • Cardia: perigastric, periesophageal, celiac, splenic, pancreaticoduodenal, and porta hepatis.
      • Body: perigastric, celiac, splenic, suprapancreatic, pancreaticoduodenal, and porta hepatis.
      • Antrum/pylorus: perigastric, celiac, suprapancreatic, pancreaticoduodenal, and porta hepatis.

Unresectable

- GTV
  - Primary tumor + clinically positive LN seen on planning CT (>1 cm short axis diameter).
    - Endoscopy reports may help determine tumor location.
    - IV contrast will aid in the definition of nodal volumes.
    - Oral contrast (5 minutes prior to simulation) aids in the definition of GTV.
    - MRI or PET fusion may aid in volume definition.
- CTV
  - Entire stomach (include 5 cm of normal esophagus for GEJ lesions).
  - Lymph node regions depending on location as for adjuvant therapy.
  - Recommend treatment with an empty stomach to reduce target volume and CTV variation within set fields. Daily image guidance for confirmation is strongly suggested in this setting.
  - PTV = CTV + 1 cm, may be reduced to 0.5 cm with daily image guidance

Treatment Planning

- Conventional 2-field
  - AP/PA arrangement preferred because it provides the best coverage of CTV and respects normal tissue tolerances.
  - Consider lateral field use in patients with anterior gastric location or when AP/PA fields cannot meet normal tissue constraints.
- 3DCRT (Figure 7.3)
  - As needed to achieve normal tissue constraints of kidneys, spinal cord, and liver, particularly when total dose is greater than 45 Gy.

FIGURE 7.3 A 59-year-old man with resected gastric adenocarcinoma, negative margins, 4-involved LN, and soft tissue involvement beyond the serosa. EBRT plan: 3-field coplanar beam arrangement (a) was chosen to limit dose to the liver and kidney. The initial fields (b) covered the regional lymph nodes (green) and the tumor bed (red).

Dose/Fractionation

- For adjuvant therapy, the CTV should receive 45 Gy/1.8 Gy/fx. May consider from 5.4 to 9 Gy boost for positive margins/gross residual disease, as determined by constraints.
- For definitive therapy, the dose to CTV is 45 Gy/1.8 Gy/fx and the GTV total dose is 54 to 59.4 Gy/1.8 Gy/fx.

RECTAL CANCER

Indications

- The once-common postoperative EBRT for resected rectal cancer is being replaced by use of neoadjuvant chemoradiotherapy.
- Concurrent chemoradiotherapy in the definitive setting, a rare scenario.

Localization, Immobilization, and Simulation

- Immobilization and patient position
  - Prone with arms above the head.
  - Consider belly board to displace small bowel.
  - Simulate and treat with full bladder to displace small bowel.
- Contrast agents and markers
  - Oral contrast to delineate the small bowel.
  - Barium enema to delineate the tumor (caution with respect to tumor displacement).
  - IV contrast to delineate the tumor and LN.
  - Anal marker to delineate the anus.
- If possible, simulate with full bladder to reduce volume of small bowel in treatment portal

Target Volume Definition

- GTV
  - Primary tumor + clinically positive nodes greater than 1 cm short axis diameter.
  - PET or MRI fusion typically aides in GTV delineation.
  - Colonoscopy reports may help determine tumor location.
- CTV
  - LN at risk for T1 to T3 tumors, include common iliac, internal iliac, and presacral LN as well as the entire mesorectum.
  - Mesorectum
    - Given variations in bladder and rectal filling, expand mesorectal coverage 1 cm anteriorly into the bladder/vagina/prostate.

- For T4 tumors, also include coverage of external iliac LN.
- If the anus, skin, or distal one third of the vagina is involved, also include inguinal LN.
- PTV
  - PTV = CTV + 1 cm

Treatment Planning

- Conventional 3-field technique (PA + opposed laterals; Figure 7.4)

FIGURE 7.4 A 49-year-old man with locally advanced rectal adenocarcinoma, stage T4N1M0, treated preoperatively with chemoradiotherapy. The initial PA (a) and lateral fields (b) covered the primary tumor (red) as well as the internal iliac (green), external iliac (green), presacral (green), and mesorectal (blue) LN. The cone down posterior (c) and lateral fields (d) covered the primary tumor and clinically involved LN (red) with margin.

- Beam weighing typically 2:1:1 for PA and laterals
  - High energy for PA field
  - 6 MV photons for laterals unless wide separation
- PA field
  - Inferior border: 3 cm below the anal marker
  - Superior border: L5/S1 vertebral body interspace
  - Lateral borders: 1.5 cm on pelvic brim or CTV, whichever is larger
- Lateral fields
  - Superior/inferior borders: same as PA field
  - Anterior border
    - T3 tumors: behind the pubic symphysis
    - T4 tumors: in front of the pubic symphysis to include external iliac LN
    - Posterior border: 1 cm behind the sacrum to include presacral lymph nodes
- Boost field: 2 cm block margin on the GTV
- Inguinal fields: see "Anal Cancer" section
- Consider IMRT for cases that require inguinal nodal coverage (better skin-sparing) and if adequate small bowel sparing is not achieved with a 3D plan.

Volumetric Planning Goals

- 95% of the PTV should receive at least 95% of the prescription dose.
- No portion of the PTV should receive less than 90% of the prescription dose.
- 99% of the CTV should receive at least 95% of the prescription dose.
- 0.1 cc of tissue is limited to 115% of the prescription dose.
- 1.0 cc of tissue (or 5% of the PTV) is limited to 110% of the prescription dose.
- 5 cc of tissue (or 10% of the PTV) is ideally limited to 105% of the prescription dose.
- See "General Principles" section for critical structure dose constraints.

Dose/Fractionation

- Chemoradiotherapy: CTV to 45 Gy/1.8 Gy/fx, boost GTV and presacral LN by additional 5.4 Gy/1.8 Gy/fx

ANAL CANCER

Introduction

- Primary management of anal cancer is definitive chemoradiotherapy.
  - Treatment for rare T1N0M0 lesions may include en face electron therapy, interstitial brachytherapy, or contact therapy.
  - Surgery is reserved for failure to achieve complete response or for local failures.

Localization, Immobilization, and Simulation

- Immobilization and patient position
  - Supine with arms across the chest or prone in a belly board in an alpha-cradle or other immobilization device, arms extended. If using the prone setup for primary fields, may consider supine positioning for the boost (which is typically away from small bowel) so that desquamated patients may be positioned more comfortably.
- Contrast agents and markers
  - Oral contrast to delineate the small bowel.
  - Barium enema to delineate the tumor.
  - IV contrast to delineate the tumor and LN.
  - Anal marker to delineate the anus.
  - Wire to involved inguinal LN.

Target Volume Definitions

- GTV
  - Primary tumor + clinically positive LN seen on planning CT (>1 cm short axis diameter).
  - PET or MRI fusion typically aides in GTV delineation.
  - Colonoscopy/anoscopy reports may help determine tumor location.
- CTV
  - LN at risk include common iliac, external iliac, internal iliac, presacral, mesorectal, perianal, and inguinal.
    - For low-lying anal lesions, inclusion of the superior portion of the mesorectum is controversial.
  - CTV = 2.5 cm expansion on primary tumor and 1 cm expansion on involved nodes
- PTV
  - PTV = CTV + 1 cm

Treatment Planning

- Conventional 2-field technique (AP/PA; Figure 7.5)
- Initial field borders
  - Superior border: L5/S1 vertebral body interspace.
  - Inferior border: 2.5 to 3 cm below the anal marker (or 3 cm margin on extent of disease if extending into the anal margin/perianal skin).
  - Lateral border
    - PA: 1.5 cm on pelvic brim.
    - AP: include inguinal nodes with 2 cm lateral to greater sciatic notch.

FIGURE 7.5 A 49-year-old woman with T3N0 squamous cell carcinoma (SCC) of the anus treated with definitive concurrent chemoradiotherapy using a 9-field IMRT approach with 10 MV photons. Prescribed 45 Gy to the regional nodes and 54 Gy to the primary tumor volume. (a) Axial, (b) sagittal, (c) coronal images displaying isodose distributions and (d) beam arrangement. Lower image (e) shows the dose-volume histogram (DVH) of the treatment plan.

- Supplement AP photon field with electrons matched to the divergence of the PA field.
- Place bolus on palpable inguinal nodes.
- In vivo dosimetry (eg, thermoluminescent dosimetry) can help determine the appropriate electron supplement.

- Cone down no. 1 field borders
  - Lower superior border to the bottom of SI joints.
  - Inferior and lateral borders remain the same.
- Boost field
  - Indicated for T3, T4, N+, or T2 lesions with residual disease after 45 Gy.
  - Use 2 cm margin on GTV via AP/PA, 3-field (opposed laterals and PA – lowest anterior skin dose), or 4-field (AP/PA/laterals) approach.
  - Alternatively, may use en face perineal electron or photon field with the patient in a frog-leg position depending on the depth of the primary tumor.
- Specific clinical scenarios may favor a 4-field technique: This usually requires higher electron supplement to the inguinal nodes, which can result in greater inguinal desquamation.
- IMRT is the evolving standard. Shrinking field or dose-painting technique may be employed. RTOG 0529 treatment volumes and doses are described below.

Volumetric Planning Goals

- 95% of the PTV should receive at least 95% of the prescription dose.
- No portion of the PTV should receive less than 85% of the prescription dose.
- 99% of the CTV should receive at least 95% of the prescription dose.
- 0.1 cc of tissue is limited to 115% of the prescription dose.
- 1.0 cc of tissue (or 5% of the PTV) is limited to 110% of the prescription dose.
- 5 cc of tissue (or 10% of the PTV) is ideally limited to 105% of the prescription dose.
- See "General Principles" section for critical structure dose constraints.
  - For external genitalia, attempt to limit
    - 50% to less than 20 Gy
    - 95% to less than 40 Gy
  - For iliac crest, may attempt to limit
    - 50% to less than 30 Gy
    - 95% to less than 50 Gy

Dose/Fractionation

- CTV to 45 Gy/1.8 Gy/fx
  - Field reduction to cone down no. 1 after 30.6 Gy.
- T3, T4, or T2 lesions with residual disease after 45 Gy should receive an additional 9 to 14.4 Gy to the GTV via boost field.
  - T2 dose goal, 45 to 50.4 Gy
  - T3 dose goal, 54 Gy
  - T4 dose goal, 54 to 59.4 Gy
- Clinically negative inguinal LN should receive a minimum of 36 Gy, measuring prescription depth on CT classically, 3 cm has been used (this may underdose thicker patients).

- Clinically positive inguinal LN should receive a minimum of 45 Gy.
  - Boost additional 5.4 to 9 Gy depending on LN size and clinical response.
- Clinically positive pelvic LN may be boosted along with primary boost field for an additional 5.4 to 9 Gy above 45 Gy CTV dose depending on LN size and clinical response.
  Per RTOG 0529 (employs IMRT using dose-painting technique):
  - For T2N0:
    - PTVA (primary tumor): 50.4 Gy in 28 fx (1.8 Gy/fx)
    - Nodal PTV: 42 Gy in 28 fx (1.5 Gy/fx)
  - For T3/4 N0:
    - PTVA (primary tumor): 54 Gy in 30 fx (1.8 Gy/fx)
    - Nodal PTV: 45 Gy in 30 fx (1.5 Gy/fx)
  - For N+:
    - PTVA (primary tumor): 54 Gy in 30 fx (1.8 Gy/fx)
    - Nodal PTV (uninvolved nodes): 45 Gy in 30 fx (1.5 Gy/fx)
    - Nodal PTV ($\leq$3 cm): 50.4 Gy in 30 fx (1.68 Gy/fx)
    - Nodal PTV (>3 cm): 54 Gy in 30 fx (1.8 Gy/fx)

STEREOTACTIC BODY RADIOTHERAPY (SBRT) FOR LIVER TUMORS

SBRT Indications

- Oligometastatic disease to the liver in selected patients
- Medically inoperable or surgically unresectable primary liver cancers

Special Considerations at Simulation

- Rigid immobilization with bodyfix device
- Compensation for respiratory movement
  - Tumor range of motion to be kept to less than 5 to 10 mm. A variety of techniques can be used to control or account for motion:
    - Active breath control (ABC)
    - Gating
    - Abdominal compression
- Tri-phase CT scan with delayed IV contrast needed to aid in delineation of GTV (native, arterial, and venous phases)
- Gold fiducial seeds may be placed prior to simulation to facilitate IGRT

Target Volume Definitions

- GTV = defined by IV contrasted CT or MRI simulation scan
  - Diagnostic MRI or PET can be fused to planning scan to aid in identification of GTV
  - CTV = GTV (for liver metastases) or + 4 to 5 mm for primary liver tumors

- ▪ ITV = target representing the range of GTV motion through the breathing cycle
  - ▪ PTV = CTV (or ITV) + 5 to 10 mm margin. Expansion will reflect the parameters of the particular delivery system, tumor motion control, and dose planning algorithm. Uniform margins are used for ITV approach, otherwise greater margin should be given cranio-caudally than in the radial aspect.

Treatment Planning

- ▪ Based mainly on single and multi-institutional experiences.
  - ▪ IMRT or dynamic conformal arcs are most often used (Figure 7.6).

FIGURE 7.6 A 48-year-old woman with a single liver metastasis from colon cancer in the posterior medial aspect of the right hepatic lobe. This lesion was treated with 45 Gy in 3 fx using two 6 MV VMAT arcs prescribed to 75% plan. (a) Axial image displaying isodose distribution. (b) Co-registered simulation and localization scans confirming proper patient position prior to treatment delivery. Lower image (c) shows the DVH of the treatment plan.

- General goals of planning:
  - Delineation of normal abdominal structures.
  - All organs at risk to have detailed dose constraints, defined by both maximum point dose and by volume.
  - Dose constraints will vary with fractionation schedule.
  - Coverage of at least 95% of the PTV by prescription isodose curve.
  - Most common constraint used: $\geq$700 mL of normal liver receiving $\leq$15 Gy.

Dose/Fractionation

- Several dose-fraction schemes have been used. Single-fraction regimens have used 18 to 30 Gy, but generally doses between 30 to 60 Gy in 3 to 5 fx are used.
- Factors to be considered in selecting prescription dose include: normal liver reserve, tumor location, and treatment intent, among others.

REFERENCE

1. http://www.rtog.org/ClinicalTrials/ProtocolTable/StudyDetails.aspx?study=0529 (accessed May 27, 2014).

8   Genitourinary Radiotherapy

Edward W. Jung, Rahul D. Tendulkar,
and Kevin L. Stephans

GENERAL PRINCIPLES

- Common principles when approaching radiation therapy planning for patients with genitourinary (GU) cancers include definition of dose-limiting structures, dose constraints, and treatment planning principles.

Localization, Immobilization, and Simulation

- Volumetric treatment planning with computed tomography [CT] simulation is recommended for all GU external beam radiation therapy (EBRT) cases.
- CT simulation with at least 3 mm axial slice acquisition.
- Patient preparation, position, and immobilization differ by disease site. Please refer to the pertinent sections.

Image Guidance for Localization and Daily Treatment Verification

- Image-guided radiation therapy (IGRT) options include cone beam CT (CBCT), ultrasound, or implanted fiducials. Hip prosthesis may limit the use of CBCT due to artifact.
- Selection of image guidance methods depends on patient factors and availability. Planning target volume (PTV) margin may be affected by type of IGRT used.

Target Volumes and Organs of Interest Definition

- Normal anatomy routinely identified (Table 8.1).
    - Small bowel: contour potential small bowel space within proximity to the PTV (suggested, 5 cm).
    - Rectum: begin contouring inferiorly at the level of the anal verge to the level of the rectosigmoid junction superiorly. The rectum is approximately 15 cm in length.
    - Bladder: contour the bladder from the level of the urachus to the bladder neck at the level of prostate.
    - Prostate: begin contouring at the level of the bladder neck and extend the contour inferiorly to the level of the prostate apex. The prostate apex is located about 1 cm above the urethrogram beak. When available, consider using MRI to define the prostate apex.
    - Penile bulb: located just inferiorly to the beak on a urethrogram.
- Seminal vesicles (as needed): contour the proximal 1 to 2 cm for intermediate and high risk prostate cancer. Consider treating the entire seminal vesicles if grossly involved.
- Femoral head/necks: contour the left and right separately, beginning at the top of the femoral head superiorly and extending inferiorly to the level of the lesser trochanters bilaterally.
- Lymph nodes (as needed; Figure 8.1) (1): start contouring at the level of L5/S1 for most GU sites as described. See also the Radiation Therapy Oncology Group (RTOG) contouring atlas.
    - Common iliac: contour from L5/S1 to the bifurcation of the external and internal iliac arteries.
    - Internal iliac: contour the internal iliacs inferiorly to the level of the prostate.
    - External iliac: contour the external iliacs inferiorly to the level of the top of the femoral heads bilaterally, at the level of the inguinal ligament.
    - Presacral: contour between S1 and S3.
    - Obturator: contour between the levels of the femoral heads superiorly to the superior-most portion of the pubis symphysis inferiorly.
- Testicles (as needed): right and left separately.
- Penis (as needed): starting at the level of penile bulb and including the corpus spongiosum, corpus cavernosum, penile shaft, and glans penis

FIGURE 8.1 Example of ports used for a 4-field box technique to treat pelvic lymph nodes. AP projection (a) and right lateral projection (b).

Treatment Planning

External beam radiation therapy with 3-dimensional conformal radiotherapy (3DCRT) planning or intensity-modulated radiation therapy (IMRT) with daily IGRT is preferred. Quality assurance for IMRT should be accomplished using phantom measurements prior to the start of treatment. Brachytherapy can be used in particular cases such as prostate cancer and select penile and urethral cases.

Lymph node (LN) irradiation

- LN irradiation is routinely used for early-stage testicular cancers, bladder cancers, high-risk prostate cancers, and advanced penile cancers.
- Clinical target volume (CTV) = 7 mm around the pertinent vessels of regional lymph node coverage depending on disease site. Exclude bone, bowel, bladder, and muscle (1).
- PTV = 5 mm around the CTV with daily image guidance

Technical Factors

Beam energies

- Photon energies 6 MV to 10 MV are typical, especially if IMRT is used. Higher-energy beams can be used in testicular cancer and for the posterior-anterior (PA) beams for penile and urethral cancer to achieve better dose homogeneity with treatment planning.

Beam shaping

■ Multileaf collimation or individually shaped (5 half value layer (HVL)) custom blocks for normal tissue protection outside the target volume are routinely used.

EXTERNAL BEAM RADIOTHERAPY FOR PROSTATE CANCER

External Beam Radiotherapy Indications

■ Intact prostate alone or combined with brachytherapy
■ Postprostatectomy in the adjuvant or salvage setting

Localization, Immobilization, and Simulation

■ Patient preparation: full bladder and empty rectum minimizes dose to critical structures (bladder, small bowel, rectum).
■ Patient position: supine, with arms folded on the chest.
■ Immobilization:
  ■ Consider a body mold such as a vacuum-lock immobilization bag.
  ■ A knee bolster with the feet banded together provides a comfortable and reproducible position.
■ Simulation: CT scan from midabdomen to midfemur.
■ CT should include the L4-L5 intervertebral disk level superiorly to below the lesser trochanters inferiorly.
■ Contrast agents may be considered:
  ■ Intravenous contrast to help delineate major blood vessels, nearby lymph nodes, and prostate-bladder interface (median lobe).
  ■ Retrograde urethrogram: 10 cc urethral contrast with penile clamp to delineate the urethra and penile bulb.
  ■ Oral contrast to delineate the small bowel.
■ If available, MRI fusion with T2 weighted scans provides the best soft tissue resolution of the prostate apex, extraprostatic extension, seminal vesicle invasion, and penile bulb.

Target Volume Definition for EBRT: Intact Prostate

■ Definition of the GTV.
  ■ There is no GTV for prostate cancer with CT-based imaging because CT is unable to define gross tumor within the gland.
  ■ GTV can sometimes be delineated using MRI.
  ■ Clinically positive nodes (>1.5 cm short axis diameter) seen on planning CT or on MRI should be included as nodal GTV.
■ Definition of the CTV.

- CTV = entire prostate +/- seminal vesicles +/- LN.
  - Low-risk prostate cancer CTV − entire prostate only.
  - Intermediate-risk prostate cancer CTV = prostate + proximal 1 cm of the bilateral seminal vesicles.
  - High-risk prostate cancer CTV = prostate + proximal 2 cm of the bilateral seminal vesicles (consider entire seminal vesicles if grossly involved) +/- LN regions.
- Definition of the PTV
  - PTV margin depends on the immobilization technique and the particular IGRT technology being used.
  - With Calypso (see below) localization and real-time tracking, a 5 to 6 mm expansion is used except posteriorly at the prostate/rectum interface where a 3 to 5 mm margin is used.
  - With CBCT IGRT, an 8 to 10 mm expansion is used, except posteriorly, where a 5 to 8 mm margin is used. The PTV expands into the rectum, whereas the CTV does not.
  - With ultrasound (U/S) IGRT, larger margins are recommended due to systematic displacement of the prostate due to probe pressure and interuser variability (2): 8 to 12 mm all around the prostate and 5 to 10 mm posterior to the prostate.

Lymph Node Irradiation (LNI)

- LNI is not standard for low- or intermediate-risk prostate cancer. LNI is controversial for high-risk prostate cancer, and is the subject of RTOG 0924.
- LN CTV = 7 mm expansion around internal/external iliac vessels, obturators, and presacral regions.
- If using 2D planning, 4-field box (Figure 8.1a and b) approach with field borders as follows:
- Anterior and posterior field:
  - Superior: L5/S1 or mid-sacroiliac (SI) joint depending on the extent of common iliac lymph node coverage.
  - Inferior: bottom of ischial tuberosity or 1.5 cm below the apex of the urethrogram.
  - Lateral: 1 to 1.5 cm lateral to the pelvic brim.
  - Block regions including the small bowel, femoral head, and external genitalia.
- Lateral field borders:
  - Anterior: 1 cm anterior to the pubic symphysis.
  - Posterior: S3/S4.
  - Block regions including the small bowel, femoral head, and external genitalia.

■ As an alternative to 2D planning, IMRT provides superior sparing of normal tissues. For lymph node coverage, see section on Target Volumes and Organs of Interest. Treatment planning for IMRT is discussed in the planning section.

Dose/Fractionation

■ Total prescription dose of 75.6 to 79.2 Gy in 1.8 to 2 Gy/fx
  ■ If treating LN prescribe initial 45 to 50.4 Gy/1.8 Gy/fx to the pelvis (lymph nodes + prostate + seminal vesicles). Grossly positive lymph nodes can be boosted to a higher dose.
    • Boost the seminal vesicles to 54 to 66 Gy, pay attention to small bowel position and potential for toxicity, and boost the prostate alone to final prescription dose.
■ A hypofractionated regimen of 70 Gy/2.5 Gy/fx may be considered. Other hypofractionated schedules include 70.2 Gy/2.7 Gy/fx, 62 Gy/3.1 Gy/fx (4 fx/week), or 51.6 Gy/4.3 Gy/fx.
■ An extremely hypofractionated regimen such as 36.25 Gy/7.25 Gy/fx (every other day), using stereotactic body radiation therapy (SBRT) may be considered. Please refer to Prostate SBRT section.

Image Guidance

■ IGRT technologies include U/S, megavoltage and kilovoltage CBCT, implanted transponders with radiofrequency emission (Calypso), and implanted gold seed fiducial markers.
■ IGRT reduces systematic errors due to rectal distention and changes in bladder filling, and provides better target localization compared with surface skin marks or bony landmarks.

Planning

Organs containing contrast are manually assigned water density during heterogeneity calculation. Plan optimization is performed to the PTV via step-and-shoot IMRT or volumetric modulated arc therapy (VMAT). Static beam IMRT using 5 beams are arranged at 0°, 50°, 100°, 260°, and 310°. This arrangement prevents aiming through the rails of the table, which can cause attenuation of the beam on some treatment machines. Lateral fields are to be avoided if a hip prosthesis is noted. Instead, anterior oblique or posterior obliques are used. Use of PA fields is avoided to minimize dose to the rectum. VMAT can be conducted with two full arcs typically employing a 90 degree collimator rotation between arcs, and can decrease overall treatment time compared to multiple static IMRT beams.

The target coverage goal is for 100% of the prescription dose to cover 95% or more of the PTV, and 99% or more of the CTV. 10 MV photon beams can provide better homogeneity than 6 MV beams, though the effect is reduced by increasing the number of beams. Hot spots should not be located in or near the rectal wall. Hot spots elsewhere are typically maintained below 107% of the prescribed dose, though this is less critical if they do not fall in sensitive tissues.

Critical Structures and Suggested Dose Constraints

Standard fractionation: See Table 8.1. Of note, IMRT plans generally allow for tighter constraints than those listed in Table 8.1, which should be considered maximum acceptable standards.

Hypofractionation (70 Gy in 2.5 Gy/fx) constraints per RTOG 0415 as follows:

- Rectum:
  - <15%, >74 Gy.
  - <25%, >69 Gy.
  - <35%, >64 Gy.
  - <50%, >59 Gy.
- Bladder:
  - <15%, >79 Gy.
  - <25%, >74 Gy.
  - <35%, >69 Gy.
  - <50%, >64 Gy.
- Femoral heads: same as conventional fractionation
- Penile bulb: mean dose <51 Gy.

Target Volume Definition for EBRT: Post-Prostatectomy

- Definition of prostate bed CTV (Figure 8.2a and b).
  - CTV = prostate bed +/- remnant seminal vesicles.
  - Contour the prostate bed inferiorly to below the urethrogram beak and continue to the top of the pubic symphysis.
  - Extend the contours laterally to the medial edge of the sacrorectogenitopubic fascia bilaterally. Where this fascia is not visible one may alternately use the medial border of the obturator internus.
  - Anteriorly include the bladder up to the pubic symphysis with gradual reduction posteriorly and superiorly to the bladder for 1 to 2 cm above the pubic symphysis.
  - Include at least 1 cm of the posterior bladder in the CTV. Extend more superiorly for patients with pathological involvement of the prostate base or seminal vesicles.

TABLE 8.1 Summary of Contouring Guidelines and Dose Constraints for Intact Prostate Using Standard Fraction Sizes of 1.8 to 2.0 Gy/fraction

Organ	Contouring Guideline	Dose Constraint	Comments
Rectum	A. Begin contouring superiorly at level of rectosigmoid junction. Continue contouring inferiorly to the level of the anal verge. B. Alternatively start at the anal verge and contour superiorly for a maximal length of 15 cm or until boundary of the rectosigmoid junction.	1. >75 Gy to ≤15% volume 2. **>70 Gy to ≤25% volume** 3. >65 Gy to ≤35% volume 4. >60 Gy to ≤50% volume Ideal: V70	Consider placing marker at anal verge. Postoperative dose constraints may be lowered if clinically indicated.
Bladder	Contour bladder from top of bladder at the level of urachus inferiorly to the bladder neck located at the level of the prostate	1. >80 Gy to ≤15% volume 2. **>75 Gy to ≤25% volume** 3. ≥70 Gy to ≤35% volume	Keep bladder full if treating bladder primary, else partly full if treating other primaries
Bowel	Contour potential bowel space beginning at L5-S1 inferiorly to the rectosigmoid junction	1. <50 Gy to ≤66% volume 2. <40 Gy to ≤100% volume	
Femoral heads	Contour left and right separately beginning at the top of the femoral head within the acetabulum and extending inferiorly to the level to the lesser trochanter bilaterally	≤10% each receive ≤50 Gy. **Keep mean dose below 45 Gy**	
Penile bulb	Located at the level of urethral beak on a urethrogram	Mean dose <52.5 Gy	Consider using MRI for better definition

■ Include the area between the bladder and rectum as well as the proximal 2 cm of the remnant seminal vesicles. The rectum should not be included in the CTV. Consider including entire seminal vesicles (SV) if SVs or the prostatic base is pathologically involved. The superior contour should be at or above the level of the vas deferens.

FIGURE 8.2 Postoperative prostate and seminal vesicle bed contour (a) and dose-volume histogram (b).

- Include surgical clips around the prostate bed. Do not include hemostasis clips higher in the pelvis if the seminal vesicles are uninvolved.
- Definition of the PTV.
  - PTV = 7 to 10 mm around the CTV. Posteriorly toward the rectum, the margin may be reduced to 5 mm.
  - Tighter margins may be used with more advanced IGRT and immobilization.

Dose/Fractionation

- Doses of 64.8 to 70.2 Gy in 1.8 to 2 Gy per fx are used postoperatively.
- A distinction can be made between adjuvant (absence of detectable disease) and salvage (presence of detectable disease) as follows:
  - 64 to 66 Gy for adjuvant therapy.

- 70 Gy for salvage therapy.
  - 45 to 50.4 Gy to pelvic lymph nodes if indicated
- Dose-volume constraints per RTOG 0534 for postprostatectomy radiation as follows:
  - Rectum:
    - <25%, >65 Gy.
    - <45%, >40 Gy.
  - Bladder:
    - <40%, >65 Gy.
    - <60%, >40 Gy.
  - Femoral heads: same as conventional fractionation.
  - Penile bulb: same as conventional fractionation.

PROSTATE BRACHYTHERAPY

Indications

- Definitive treatment for low- or intermediate-risk patients.
- Combination treatment with external beam radiation therapy.

Patient Evaluation

- Determining which patients are good candidates for prostate brachytherapy is highly operator/institutional dependent and relies on the skill and experience of the treating physician.
- Volume study with U/S may be used. Ideal volume is <60 cc per American Brachytherapy Society recommendations; larger glands are implanted successfully at select centers.
- Evaluate pubic arch interference with CT or U/S.
- If prostate volume is too large or pubic arch interference exists, hormone therapy can be initiated 2 to 3 months prior to implantation for gland size reduction if needed before prostate brachytherapy resulting in less likelihood of urinary obstructive complications.

Setup and Preparation (Figure 8.3)

- Preoperatively, patients are instructed to avoid aspirin and anticoagulants for at least 5 days.
- Fleet enema is given on the morning of the procedure.
- Perioperative intravenous antibiotics such as cefazolin 1 gram (2 grams for patients >70 kg), or ciprofloxacin if penicillin allergic, are recommended.
- Gentamycin 80 mg coverage is added if a patient has a metal implant or a pacemaker.

FIGURE 8.3 Patient setup and preparation for prostate brachytherapy.

- General (or spinal) anesthesia is used.
- Patient is placed in an extended dorsal lithotomy position.
- Patient positioning is critical to minimize pubic bone interference during seed placement. Pelvis must be flexed so the pubic arch is elevated.
- The genitalia are taped anteriorly out of the field, the perineal skin is shaved, and the rectum is irrigated with saline and a rectal catheter.
- The perineum is prepped with betadine.
- 10 cc of ultrasound jelly is injected into the rectum.
- A U/S probe is placed within the rectum using a U/S stabilization device.
- The U/S stabilization device helps ensure reproducibility from the time of initial U/S image acquisition and treatment planning to final seed insertion.
- Minimize readjustment of the U/S stabilization device after a treatment plan has been finalized, as this could lead to a geometric miss during seed insertion.

Technique (Figure 8.4)

- Radioactive ^{125}I (Iodine-125; T½ = 60 days, 28 keV photon), ^{109}Pd (Palladium-109; T½ = 17 days, 21 keV photon), or ^{131}I (Cesium-131; T½ = 9.7 days, 29 keV photon) seeds are commonly used.
- Transrectal US (TRUS) images of the prostate are captured at 5 mm intervals and exported to a treatment planning system.
- Treatment planning can be accomplished preoperatively or intraoperatively.
- Before image acquisition, one should ensure that the prostatic urethra is midline. There should be minimum pubic bone interference using an exaggerated dorsal lithotomy position (Figure 8.3).
- Measure the prostate height, width, length, and volume. These measurements are used for 2 purposes:

FIGURE 8.4 Isodose distribution (a), number of seeds/needle (b), prostate dose-volume histogram (c), and sagittal ultrasound (d) to guide seed placement.

■ The number of longitudinal images acquired at 0.5 cm intervals should correspond with the length of the prostate (eg, a length of 4.5 cm should yield 8 to 10 axial images for planning, whereas 9 would be an exact match: 4.5 cm/0.5 cm = 9). The subtle differences in the number images planes acquired are due to volume averaging effects.

- The algorithms used by most commercially available U/S machines calculate volume using the following equation: ([length × width × height] × 0.52).
  - This approach differs from that used by most treatment planning systems in which the series of volumes of slices 0.5 cm thick are added together. Having two independently calculated volumes that agree within 10% of each other adds confidence in the image acquisition and contouring process.
- Commercial planning software is used for contouring the prostate on each slice and for placing seeds within the contoured prostate (Figure 8.4a).
- Stranded or linked sources are placed peripherally. Loose seeds are placed centrally because they are easier to remove as a single source cystoscopically and spontaneously if misplaced or if placed within the urethra or the bladder.
- The urethra can be visualized on the TRUS. Use of a Foley catheter or injected contrast is typically not needed and often obstructs the view of the anterior part of the prostate. Ensure that the urethra is located at the midline of the template (ie, the "D" line in this case) because this helps to minimize the risk of seed placement within the urethra.
- If urethral visualization is inadequate, consider injecting 3 to 5 ml mixture of lubricant jelly and air or place a Foley catheter +/- contrast. Of note, this may lead to shadowing artifacts anteriorly.
- Image acquisition and physics planning may be done preoperatively or intraoperatively.
- A final plan will display the number of needles, the number of sources, and the exact geometric location where the needles should be inserted (Figure 8.4b).
- Preplan goals as follows:
  - Volume receiving 100% of dose (V100) = 100%.
  - Volume receiving 150% of dose (V150) ≤50%.
  - Volume receiving 200% of dose (V200) ≤20%.
  - Dose to 90% of prostate should be around 115% to 120%.
  - Central prostatic (urethral) dose should be <150% of planned dose.
- A final dose-volume histogram (DVH) should be analyzed to ensure that it meets the specified goal (Figure 8.4c).
- Radioactive seeds are loaded into needles according to the plan.
- The number of seeds needed is usually around 80 to 120 for ^{125}I but can vary significantly depending on the volume of the gland, the geometry of the implant, the prescription dose, and the source activity.
- Figure 8.5 shows the total implant activity versus prostate volume. Using this graph as a general guideline for the brachytherapy plan helps reduce potential prescription errors (eg, if the total prescription dose was not set properly, the plan will not plot in the area of the graph consistent with its volume-activity ratio).

FIGURE 8.5 Prostate volume versus total activity.

- The needles are then inserted into the perineum under U/S guidance.
- Start placement of needles in the axial coordinate farthest from the TRUS probe to minimize image distortion during seed placement.
- One should pay close attention to the rectal-prostate interface at the prostate apex during needle placement to minimize risk for seed placement within the rectum (Figure 8.4d).
- Cystoscopy is indicated if gross blood is present at the urethral meatus and does not clear with bladder irrigation.
- Survey meter reading at 1 meter from patient must be less than 1 millirem per hour (1 mR/h) for the patient to be discharged for I-125 and Pd-103.
- Survey meter measurements are also taken on contact with patient surface and at 10 cm distance from the patient.

Target Volume Definition for Postimplant Prostate Brachytherapy Assessment

- Definition of CTV:
  - CTV = prostate for low risk.
  - CTV = prostate + 0.5 to 1 cm of the proximal seminal vesicles for intermediate and high risk.
  - Contour the prostate on each slice at 5 mm intervals.
- Definition of the PTV:

- PTV = CTV + 5 to 8 mm inferiorly, 5 mm superiorly, 3 mm anteriorly, zero margin posteriorly. Margins may vary based on institutional preference. However, there should never be a posterior PTV margin expansion into the rectum.

Postimplantation Patient Directions

- Prescribe antibiotics (ciprofloxacin 500 mg BID by mouth) for 7 to 10 days.
- Prescribe alpha-blocker (eg, tamsulosin 0.8 mg by mouth at bedtime or terazosin 5–10 mg by mouth at bedtime) for 2 to 6 months.
- Pain should be minimal after implantation. Nonsteroidal anti-inflammatory drugs (NSAIDs) may be considered for postoperative pain. If severe or persistent pain, further evaluation is required, including consideration of urine studies to rule out urinary tract infection.
- Advise that the patient return around 4 weeks postimplant for a CT scan to evaluate the quality of the seed placement.

Dose/Fractionation

- Monotherapy prescription dose is 144 to 160 Gy for ^{125}I and 115 to 125 Gy for ^{103}Pd during implantation.
- When administered as combination therapy with 45 Gy pelvis EBRT, prescription dose is 108 to 110 Gy for ^{125}I and 90 to 100 Gy for ^{103}Pd.

POSTIMPLANT DOSIMETRY

- The prostate, bladder, and rectum are contoured on each posttreatment CT image slice (Figure 8.6) to generate organ volumes (Figure 8.7a).
- Commercial planning software is then used to determine the location of each seed on the posttreatment CT.
- The location of each seed, and related reconstructed post-plan dosimetry, with respect to the contoured volumes is used to assess the quality of the intraoperative seed placement (Figure 8.7b).
- Desired dosimetric outcomes for monotherapy:
  - D90 >90% to 100%. Minimum dose to 90% of the prostate PTV (D90) should be greater than 90% to 100% of the prescribed dose.
    - V150 <70%; V150 <50% is ideal. The 150% IDL should be situated peripherally with central (urethral) sparing.
  - Ideally, 95% of the prostate volume should receive 100% of the prescribed dose (V100 >95%).
- Urethral dose should be limited to a maximum of 150% of the prescription dose.
- Volume of the rectum receiving 100% of the prescribed dose should be less than 1 to 1.3 cc, depending on the timing of the scan (3–6).

FIGURE 8.6 Postimplantation contouring for quality assurance of prostate brachytherapy.

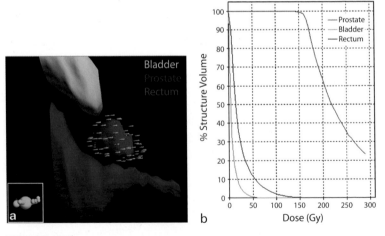

FIGURE 8.7 Postimplantation 3D rendering (a) and dose-volume histogram (b) for quality assurance of prostate brachytherapy.

PROSTATE STEREOTACTIC BODY RADIATION THERAPY (SBRT)

Indications

- Ongoing role as definitive treatment currently being defined for intact prostate cancer based on emerging outcomes data.
- Treat patients on protocol if possible (such as RTOG 0938).

Localization, Immobilization, and Simulation

- Patient preparation
    - MRI fusion may allow more accurate delineation of the CTV, though is not required. If MRI unavailable, use retrograde urethrogram to help define apex and penile bulb.
    - Fiducial markers (ie, gold seeds, Calypso) should be placed for localization.
    - Full bladder minimizes dose to small bowel and bladder.
- Simulation
    - A body mold is recommended for immobilization.
    - Rectal balloon is institution/protocol dependent, inflated with 60 to 120 cc air.
- Localization
    - IGRT must be used to accurately deliver SBRT.
- Target volume definition (as per RTOG 0938)
    - GTV = CTV defined as the prostate only on CT or MRI
        - Consider inclusion of seminal vesicles for Gleason 7 disease or higher.
    - PTV = CTV + 0 to 3 mm margin posteriorly and 3 to 5 mm in all other directions.

Dosing: variable dependent on protocol and fractionation. Typically 35 to 40 Gy administered in 5 fractions.

Critical structures and constraints are protocol dependent (eg, RTOG 0938: www.rtog.org/ClinicalTrials/ProtocolTable/StudyDetails.aspx?study=0938)

BLADDER CANCER

RT Indications

- Muscle-invasive bladder cancer.
    - Induction and consolidative chemoradiation therapy after transurethral resection of bladder tumor (TURBT).
- Nonmuscle invasive bladder cancer
    - Consider in select cases refractory to initial medical management.

Localization, Immobilization, and Simulation

- Patient position: supine with arms on chest.
- Patient preparation: bladder empty vs. full is controversial.
  - Full bladder pushes away more of the small bowel, but may vary day to day.
  - Empty bladder is more reproducible with daily treatment and minimizes treatment volume (CTV) when treating the whole bladder. Current RTOG studies and recommendations endorse empty bladder treatment.
- Full bladder volume when boosting as cone down to the tumor to minimize dose to the small bowel. If poor tumor localization due to insufficient information on bladder mapping or surgical clip placement, boost entire bladder while empty to minimize boost volume.
- Bladder fiducials (cystoscopically placed) are optional.
- The bladder wall is 0.5 to 1 cm beyond contrast on radiograph (contrast outlines inner wall of bladder).
- Immobilization: vacuum-lock immobilization is recommended.

Target Volume Definition

- Definition of the GTV
  - GTV = pre-TURBT tumor volume (as assessed on cystoscopy with bladder mapping, CT, PET, or MRI).
- Definition of the CTV
  - CTV = GTV + entire bladder + proximal urethra + prostate and prostatic urethra (in men) or proximal 2 cm of the female urethra + regional lymphatics (internal iliac, external iliac, and obturators).
  - PTV = CTV + margin (2 to 3 cm superiorly and inferiorly and 1 to 2 cm radially).
- Boost
  - CTV_{boost} = GTV + 0.5 cm
  - If GTV not well defined or lack of bladder mapping, entire bladder (empty) is CTV
  - PTV_{boost} = CTV_{boost} + 1 to 2 cm margin, depending on IGRT method used

Special Considerations

- Preinduction and postinduction cystoscopies are important for bladder and tumor mapping as well as for tumor response assessment.
- The tumor map is used for the boost portion of radiation during the consolidation phase of treatment.

Treatment Planning

- A 4-field approach is typical (Figure 8.8a and b):
  - Use AP, PA fields weighted 70% with borders as follows:

FIGURE 8.8 Four-field box technique for bladder cancer using AP/PA (a) and opposed laterals (b); bladder CTV is delineated in red.

- Superior: S2-S3 interspace. L5-S1 may be recommended if superior nodal involvement within 1 cm of S2-S3.
- Inferior border: bottom of the obturator foramen (or ischial tuberosities).
- Lateral border: 1.5 to 2 cm margin around pelvic brim, block femoral heads.

■ Use opposed lateral fields weighted 30% with borders as follows:
  ■ Superior and inferior borders same as AP/PA fields.
  ■ Anterior border: 1 to 2 cm margin on the bladder (seen as air bubble), anterior to pubic symphysis.
  ■ Posterior border: split the rectum (or 2–3 cm behind the bladder). Ensure at least 2 cm margin around CTV for anterior and posterior borders.

■ Cone down:
  ■ Repeat cystoscopy after approximately 40 Gy to pelvis to assess response for surgical candidates (no break for inoperable patients).
  ■ Cone down to tumor + 2 cm for complete responders, for a total dose of 64.8 Gy/1.8 Gy /fraction

Dose/Fractionation

■ Either once- or twice-daily regimens can be used.
■ For the BID regimen, radiation is delivered as follows:
  ■ First 5 days:
    - PTV_{pelvis}: 1.6 Gy/fx × 5 days in the morning.
    - $PTV_{bladder}$: 1.5 Gy/fx × 5 days in the evening.
  ■ Next 8 days:
    - PTV_{pelvis}: 1.6 Gy/fx × 5 days per week in the morning.
    - PTV_{boost}: 1.5 Gy/fx × 5 days per week in the evening.

- After 40.3 Gy to the tumor, patients undergo repeat cystoscopy followed by consolidative boost over 8 days as follows:
  - PTV_{pelvis}: 1.5 Gy/fx BID for a total pelvis dose of 44.8 Gy.
  - PTV_{boost}: total dose 64.3 Gy.
- The total dose of 64.3 is delivered in 42 fractions over 9 weeks.
- Once-daily radiation can be delivered as follows:
  - PTV pelvis: 1.8 to 2 Gy/fx to an initial dose of approximately 40 to 45 Gy.
  - Patient should undergo repeat cystoscopy followed by consolidative boost of 1.8 to 2 Gy/fx, for a total dose of approximately 64 Gy to PTV_{boost} and 44 Gy to PTV_{pelvis}.

Treatment Planning

- In addition to the dose constraints presented in the "General Principles" section, also consider the following:
  - 50% of the rectum should be below 55 Gy.
  - Maximum dose to the femoral heads should be limited to 45 Gy.
  - Maximum dose to the small bowel is less than 50 Gy.
- 3DCRT is used for treatment planning.
- IMRT is not standard.
- Consider wedging the lateral fields to compensate for an anterior abdominal slope.
- Multiple field arrangements may be used to optimize treatment, including 4-field, opposed lateral, and 3 to 4 oblique fields; the choice depends on physician experience, tumor location, target volume, and dose from initial large pelvic portals to dose-limiting structures such as femoral heads, rectum, and small bowel.
- Preferential weighting may aid in limiting the rectal and femoral head doses; much of the bladder is anterior, and therefore, weighing to the anterior field may be favorable.
- Weighting the AP/PA fields 70% and lateral fields 30% may spare femoral heads.
- Utilizing lateral beams for boost may spare more bladder volume.

TESTICULAR CANCER

Indications

- For early-stage (I-IIB) seminomas, external beam radiation therapy can be used adjuvantly after inguinal orchiectomy. Other options include chemotherapy alone or active surveillance. Surveillance is the preferred option for most stage I patients. EBRT is preferred for stage IIA or IIB (7–11). Full-dose chemotherapy is preferred for stage IIC and above.

- RT may also be used as salvage therapy for retroperitoneal nodal recurrence after initial chemotherapy or active surveillance.
- Tumor size >4 cm and rete testis invasion are no longer considered predictors of relapse based on a validation study and should not be used for risk-adapted management for Stage I seminoma (7).
- Relative contraindications to RT include horseshoe kidney, inflammatory bowel disease, or prior RT to the region.

Localization, Immobilization, and Simulation

- Patient-simulated supine with arms up or at sides.
- Clamshell for contralateral remaining testis. Sperm banking should be discussed prior to simulation.
- Penis should be moved out of field.
- Knee bolster can be used for patient comfort.

Target Volume Definition

Either para-aortic or "dogleg" fields are the standard for regional nodal coverage (8). Para-aortic fields are favored due to decreased toxicity at the expense of a slightly increased risk of pelvic relapse.

- "Dogleg" field should be utilized in the following scenarios:
  - Prior inguinal surgery.
  - Lymph node-positive disease (stage II).
  - If treating with RT as salvage therapy for recurrence
- 2D Planning field definition:
- Para-aortic field borders (Figure 8.9a):
  - Superior: top of T12 vertebral body. *Note: Historically, the superior border was top of T11.
  - Inferior: bottom of L5.
  - Lateral: tips of the transverse processes bilaterally. Careful attention should be paid to renal doses because wide lateral borders will result in increased dose to the kidney.
  - Include the left renal hilum for left-sided cancers. Left renal hilar nodes are usually included when left lateral border is placed at tips of the transverse processes.
- "Dogleg" field borders (Figure 8.9b):
  - Superior: top of T12 vertebral body.
  - Inferior: top of acetabulum.
  - Lateral: line from tip of the ipsilateral transverse process of L5 to the superolateral border of the ipsilateral acetabulum.
  - Medial: tip of contralateral transverse process of L5 toward the medial border of the ipsilateral obturator foramen.

FIGURE 8.9 2D-defined "dogleg" (a) and PA (b) field setup for early-stage seminoma are shown, with kidneys in teal and CTV in red. "Dogleg" field for a patient with an enlarged node using 3D planning (c) (9). Arteries are shown in red, veins in blue, with left and right kidneys in teal and orange, respectively.

- 3D Planning
  - 3D planning is preferred due to potential of marginal miss, with 2D planning based on bony anatomy (9). 3D planning improves target definition and kidney/small bowel shielding.
- Definition of the GTV for lymph node–positive disease:
  - GTVnode = positive lymph nodes seen on imaging.

- Definition of the CTV:
  - CTV = Retroperitoneal +/− ipsilateral iliac lymph node region
  - Para-aortic field: retroperitoneal lymph node coverage
    - Contour the inferior vena cava and aorta separately from 2 cm below the top of the kidneys down to the point where these vessels bifurcate.
    - Use a 1.2 cm expansion radially around the inferior vena cava and a 1.9 cm expansion around the aorta, excluding bone and bowel.
  - Dogleg field: Ipsilateral iliac lymph node coverage (Figure 8.9).
    - In addition to the para-aortic field described above, contour the ipsilateral common, external, and proximal internal iliac veins and arteries down to the upper border of the acetabulum.
    - Use a 1.2 cm expansion on the iliac vessels, excluding bone and bowel.
  - CTV_{node} = GTV_{node} + 0.8 cm, excluding bone and bowel
- Definition of the PTV:
  - PTV = CTV + 0.5 cm.
  - PTV_{node} = CTV_{node} + 0.5 cm.
  - Incorporate a 7 mm expansion around the PTVs to block edge to account for beam penumbra.

Dose/Fractionation

- 20 Gy in 2 Gy/fx is preferred or 25.5 Gy in 1.7 Gy/fx
- 20 Gy vs. 30 Gy in 2 Gy fractions demonstrates similar efficacy with reduced side effects in a randomized trial for stage I seminoma (10).
- Stage II or recurrent cancer after observation should be treated with an initial dogleg field, and then a boost should be delivered to the nodal GTV.
  - Lymph nodes ≤2 cm: boost to 30 Gy.
  - Lymph nodes between 2 and 5 cm: boost to 36 Gy.
    For lymph nodes >5 cm, bleomycin, etoposide, cisplatin (BEP) chemotherapy is the preferred treatment.
- Dose constraints
  - Kidneys: D50 ≤8, mean dose ≤9 Gy.
  - If patient has only one kidney, then D15 ≤20.
  - Boost constraints:
    - Kidneys: D50 ≤2, mean dose ≤3 Gy.

Treatment Planning

- AP/PA setup is the standard approach for all testicular cancer treatment planning fields (para-aortic, "dogleg", boost) since it delivers low dose to critical structures (kidney, liver, small bowel).
- PTV should be readily covered with the standard AP/PA setup.

- Treatment planning goal of D95 ≥100 for PTV coverage with 3D volume based planning.
- IMRT should be avoided due to higher doses to critical structures and increased integral body dose relative to an AP/PA setup, potentially increasing the risk of secondary cancers.
- Photons 10 to 18 MV allow for greater skin sparing while increasing the homogeneity of dose distribution relative to lower-energy photons.
- Antiemetic medication prophylaxis approximately 2 hours prior to treatment can improve nausea.

PENILE CANCER

Indications

- Brachytherapy or EBRT may be used for early-stage (T1, T2, and select T3) lesions in an attempt for penile preservation.
- Combined modality approach can be considered for more advanced lesions.

Brachytherapy

- Can be considered for lesions less than 4 cm with invasion of corpora cavernosa less than 1 cm.
- Typically reserved for T1, T2, and select T3 lesions
- Consider limiting brachytherapy for volume size less than 8 cc and use of less than six needles to minimize adverse effects.
- Treat full thickness of the penile shaft; clinical staging may be unreliable because it may underestimate the extent of the disease.
- Either low-dose rate (LDR) or high-dose rate (HDR) can be used.
- Place interstitial templates on each side of the penile shaft for stabilization and insertion of the needles.
- Enclose the penile shaft in a supportive styrofoam collar.
- Needles are inserted perpendicular and parallel, 1 cm apart, and typically in three planes, with two to three needles in each plane for larger lesions.
- Often, needles are inserted as a single plane of two to three needles for smaller lesions.
- Target volume is tumor plus 1.5 to 2 cm.
- Dose is 60 to 65 Gy (46–50 Gy at the center of the organ and limit urethra dose to 50 Gy).

External Beam RT

- A patient ineligible for brachytherapy based on tumor size (>4 cm), depth of invasion (>1 cm), and stage (T2 lesions >4 cm, most T3) can be considered for EBRT.

Simulation/immobilization

- Patient position: supine with arms on chest. Frog-leg position if treating the inguinal region.
- Immobilization: vacuum-lock bag.
- Techniques to immobilize the penile shaft include wax mold, Presplex block, plastic cylinder, and water bath.
- The purpose of immobilization technique is to provide dose buildup to the surface of the shaft and for reproducibility of the geometry during a course of fractionated radiotherapy.

Target definition

- Pelvic nodal irradiation can be omitted if deep pelvic lymph nodes are clinically negative.
- Treat only the involved groin if the contralateral side has been surgically staged and found to be negative, including the deep pelvic nodes.

Dose/technique

- Use parallel-opposed lateral photon beams to 45 to 50.4 Gy to the whole penile shaft, followed by a cone down to 60 to 70 Gy to 2 cm margin.
- For in situ tumor (T_{is}), consider 125 to 250 kV orthovoltage or 13 MeV electrons to 35 Gy in 10 fx of 3 to 5 Gy/fx.
- Use AP/PA to cover inguinal LN. Negative nodes should receive 50 Gy. Palpable/unresectable nodes should be treated to 70 to 75 Gy.
- Refer to the vulvar cancer treatment planning section on radiation to the inguinal region.

URETHRAL CANCER

- Management of urethral cancer with radiotherapy depends on tumor location, extent of disease, patient status, and patient sex, because surgery is the primary management tool.

Male Urethra

- Bulbomembranous urethral tumors can be treated with AP/PA fields to 45 Gy/1.8 Gy/fx, followed by a perineal and inguinal to 70 Gy if positive.
- Lesions of the prostatic urethra are treated similar to prostate cancer.
- EBRT for distal urethral cancers is similar to radiotherapy for penile cancers (see "Penile Cancer" section).
  - Interstitial brachytherapy can be considered for low-grade distal lesions measuring less than 4 cm in size at stage T1 or early T2.
    - The Memorial Hospital or Syed template can be used with a three-way Foley catheter for urine drainage, stabilization of the implant, and irrigation of the bladder if needed.

- Six needles are placed 1 cm apart around a 1 cm radius about the urethra.
- Volume of implant is tumor + 1 to 2 cm margin.
- Dose is 60 Gy with brachytherapy alone or 20 to 30 Gy combined with an EBRT dose of 45 Gy for a total dose of 65 to 75 Gy.

Female Urethra

- Early-stage lesions of the anterior distal one-third urethra:
  - May be treated with radiation therapy alone with interstitial or a combination of interstitial and EBRT.
  - Inguinal lymph nodes should be treated for more invasive disease and if clinically node positive.
- Urethral meatus carcinomas can be treated with interstitial ^{192}Ir LDR implant consisting of 8 to 12 needles arranged in an arc around the urethral orifice to a dose of 60 to 70 Gy at 0.4 Gy/h. Treatment volume is typically tumor + 1 to 2 cm.
- Posterior urethral lesions or lesions involving the entire length of the urethra have potential for bladder involvement. Thus, they should be considered for preoperative radiotherapy followed by exenterative surgery (transpubic approach is common) with inguinal lymph node dissection and urinary diversion.
- For larger tumors with extension into the labia, vagina, entire urethra, or base of the bladder:
  - Consider combined EBRT + brachytherapy implant.
  - EBRT should include the pelvic and inguinal lymph nodes in a manner analogous to vulvar/vaginal cancer treatment to a dose of 45 Gy to the whole pelvis, followed by a boost of 10 to 15 Gy to positive nodes via reduced fields. The perineum should be treated to cover the entire urethra. Please refer to the appropriate gynecological radiotherapy section for EBRT simulation and treatment planning for urethral cancer.
  - The primary site is boosted using brachytherapy via a vaginal cylinder to a dose of 60 Gy to the entire urethra.
  - An interstitial implant can then be used to further boost the tumor dose to a total dose of 70 to 80 Gy.

REFERENCES

1. Lawton CA, Michalski J, El-Naqa I, et al. RTOG GU radiation oncology specialists reach consensus on pelvic lymph node volumes for high-risk prostate cancer. *Int J Radiat Oncol Biol Phys.* 2009;74:383–387.

2. McGahan JP, Ryu J, Fogata M. Ultrasound probe pressure as a source of error in prostate localization for external beam radiotherapy. *Int J Radiat Oncol Biol Phys.* 2004;60:788–793.

3. Mueller A, Wallner K, Merrick G, et al. Perirectal seeds as a risk factor for prostate brachytherapy-related rectal bleeding. *Int J Radiat Oncol Biol Phys.* 2004;59:1047–1052.

4. Waterman FM, Dicker AP. Probability of late rectal morbidity in 125I prostate brachytherapy. *Int J Radiat Oncol Biol Phys.* 2003;55:342–353.

5. Tran A, Wallner K, Merrick G, et al. Rectal fistulas after prostate brachytherapy. *Int J Radiat Oncol Biol Phys.* 2005;63:150–154.

6. Snyder KM, Stock RG, Hong SM, et al. Defining the risk of developing grade 2 proctitis following 125I prostate brachytherapy using a rectal dose–volume histogram analysis. *Int J Radiat Oncol Biol Phys.* 2001;50:335–341.

7. Chung P, Warde P. Stage I seminoma: Adjuvant treatment is effective but is it necessary? *J Natl Cancer Inst.* 2011;103:194e–196.

8. Fossa SD, Horwich A, Russell JM, et al. Optimal planning target volume for stage I testicular seminoma: a Medical Research Council randomized trial. Medical Research Council Testicular Tumor Working Group. *J Clin Oncol.* 1999;17:1146.

9. Wilder RB, Buyyounouski MK, Efstathiou JA, et al. Radiotherapy treatment planning for testicular seminoma. *Int J Radiat Oncol Biol Phys.* 2012;83(4):e445–e452.

10. Jones WG, Fossa SD, Mead GM, et al. Randomized trial of 30 versus 20 Gy in the adjuvant treatment of stage I testicular seminoma: a report on Medical Research Council Trial TE18, European Organisation for the Research and Treatment of Cancer Trial 30942 (ISRCTN18525328). *J Clin Oncol.* 2005;23:1200–1208.

11. Bruns F, Bremer M, Meyer A, et al. Adjuvant radiotherapy in stage I seminoma: is there a role for further reduction of treatment volume? *Acta Oncol.* 2005;44:142e–148.

9   Gynecologic Radiotherapy

Rupesh R. Kotecha and Sheen Cherian

GENERAL PRINCIPLES

- Gynecologic malignancies routinely managed by radiation oncologists include endometrial, cervical, vaginal, and vulvar primary sites.
- The specific dose prescription will be determined by the tumor types and treatment approaches, eg, preoperative, definitive, postoperative, or palliative therapy.

Localization, Immobilization, and Simulation

- Volumetric treatment planning (computed tomography [CT] simulation on a flat surface) for definition of gross tumor volume (GTV), clinical target volume (CTV), and planning target volume (PTV).
- Patient position: supine or prone depending on body habitus and patient tolerance:
  - Supine position may be more reproducible.
  - Prone position with belly board may be used to displace the bowel anteriorly and superiorly.

- Immobilization with customized body mold that fixes the position of the upper body, trunk, and proximal legs.
- Consider using vaginal, anal, and cervical markers to delineate normal tissue structures.
- Contiguous spiral CT slices should be acquired with a 3 mm slice acquisition to cover the entire pelvis.
- Intravenous (IV) contrast is recommended. Oral or rectal contrast may be used (caution for anatomical distortion).
- The patient should have a full bladder during simulation and during daily radiation therapy treatments.
    - For intensity-modulated radiation therapy (IMRT) treatment planning in the definitive setting (intact uterus), two separate treatment planning CT scans with full and empty bladder should be fused before outlining the target volumes and an internal target volume (ITV) approach should be adopted.

Target Volumes and Organs of Interest Definition for Whole Pelvic Radiation

- Two-dimensional (2D) planning is based on bony anatomy.
- Conventional whole pelvic radiation therapy (WPRT) borders include (Figure 9.1)
    - Superior: L4-L5 or L5-S1 interspace.
    - Inferior: bottom of the obturator foramina to cover the proximal two-thirds of the vagina or lowest extent of disease with a 3 cm margin.
    - Lateral: 2 cm beyond the lateral margins of the true bony pelvis.

FIGURE 9.1 Conventional borders for whole pelvic radiation: (a) AP view and (b) lateral view.

- Anterior: anterior margin of the pubic symphysis.
- Posterior: through the S2-S3 interface, may extend if necessary for adequate margin.
- When extended field radiation therapy is indicated, the border should be extended superiorly to include the T12-L1 interspace.
- CT scan is used to delineate the regions of interest for 3D treatment planning.
- Lymph node group contours for WPRT include the following, using the vasculature as a surrogate (per Radiation Therapy Oncology Group [RTOG] 0418 protocol) (3):
  - Lower common iliac nodes: superior limit of the contoured common iliac will be at the top of L5 vertebral body—the PTV should be at the top of L5; therefore, the CTV should be contoured up to 7 mm from the top of L5.
  - Internal iliac nodes (obturator, inferiorly to upper third of the obturator fossa, and hypogastric).
  - External iliac nodes up to the level of the top of the femoral heads
  - Presacral nodes up to inferior border of S2.
  - PTV of 7 mm margin around the CTV.
  - Include para-aortic nodes if involved.
- Bladder: whole bladder.
- Rectum: volume to include portion inferior to the PTV and superior to level that it leaves the posterior pelvis around the region of the rectosigmoid.
- Small bowel: volume to include at least 2 cm above the PTV and the surrounding loops of small bowel out to the edge of the peritoneum.
- Femoral heads.
- Sacrum.
- ITV generated from CTV(s) outlined on the full-bladder scan and modified to include the excursion of target tissues on the empty bladder scan.

Treatment Planning

- Two (anteroposterior-posteroanterior [AP/PA]) or four (AP, PA, right lateral, and left lateral) photon fields.
- IMRT: investigational in the definitive setting, may improve normal tissue sparing in the adjuvant setting.
- 10 MV or higher energy photons are generally used.

Critical Structures

- For extended field radiation therapy:
  - Two-thirds of each kidney should not receive more than 18 Gy.
  - Dose to volume of at least 0.03 cc of the spinal cord should be limited to 45 Gy.
- Suggested dose constraints for IMRT per RTOG 0418 (3) (Table 9.1).

TABLE 9.1 Suggested Dose Constraints for Intensity-Modulated Radiation Therapy per RTOG 0418 (3)

	% Volume	Gy Constraint
Small bowel	<30	>40
Rectum	<60	>30
Bladder	<35	>45
Femoral head	<15	>30

Brachytherapy

- A variety of applicators are used, including vaginal cylinder, double tandem, tandem, and ovoids/ring.
- Common techniques:
  - High-dose rate (HDR) intracavitary implant: vaginal cylinder:
    - The patient is placed in dorsal lithotomy position.
    - A bladder catheter with balloon is placed.
    - The largest diameter cylinder that can be used is chosen (2.0–3.5 cm).
    - CT simulation in treatment position is used for volumetric planning.
  - HDR intracavitary implant: tandem and ovoids/ring:
    - Dorsal lithotomy position under sedation.
    - Radio-opaque markers are placed at the anterior and posterior lips of the cervix.
    - Bladder and rectal catheters are placed.
    - Tandem is placed at midline; colpostats/ring is symmetrically positioned against the cervix. The vagina is packed to displace the bladder and rectum; alternatively, a rectal retractor can be used.
    - CT imaging to assess applicator placement and brachytherapy planning.
  - HDR interstitial implant: Syed technique:
    - Dorsal lithotomy position under general anesthesia.
    - Radio-opaque markers are placed on the visible lesions of interest.
    - Obturator placed in the vaginal vault; the template is introduced over the obturator and made flush with the perineum.
    - Flexiguide catheters are placed into template to adequately cover the tumor volume.
    - May be done under fluoroscopic or laparoscopic guidance.
    - Template is sutured into place at four corners.
    - Patients are admitted to the hospital and the template remains in place for 2 to 3 days.
- Low-dose rate (LDR) implant may also be used for intracavitary or interstitial approaches.

ENDOMETRIAL CANCER

Indications

- Adjuvant radiation therapy for resected endometrial cancer.
- Preoperative radiation therapy: for stage IIIB tumors precluding upfront radical hysterectomy.
- Definitive radiation therapy: for medically inoperable patients or those with unresectable disease.

External Beam RT in the Adjuvant Setting

- Localization, immobilization, and simulation:
  - Per "General Principles."
- Target volumes and organs of interest definition:
  - 3D planning is recommended for full nodal coverage.
  - Per "General Principles."
  - GTV: none.
  - CTV: lymph node delineation per general principles:
    - Include all pelvic nodal regions, including presacral nodes.
    - Include the entire length of the vagina for patients with stage IIIB disease.
    - Include para-aortic nodes if involved.
  - PTV: per "General Principles."
- Treatment planning:
  - Per general principles.
- Dose:
  - For WPRT alone, use 45 to 50 Gy at 1.8 to 2 Gy/fx.
  - If brachytherapy is planned, treat with WPRT to 45 Gy.
  - Deliver 45 Gy to PA lymph nodes (LNs) if extended field is used.

Brachytherapy in the Adjuvant Setting

- General principles:
  - Given 4 to 6 weeks postoperatively or 1 week after completion of external beam radiation therapy (EBRT).
  - HDR brachytherapy is delivered with a vaginal cylinder (alternatively, colpostats may be used).
- Localization, immobilization, and simulation:
  - HDR intracavitary implant: vaginal cylinder per "General Principles."
- Target volumes and organs of interest definition:
  - Treat the proximal 4 cm of the vagina.
  - Consider treating the entire length of the vagina for stage IIIB disease.
  - Contour the bladder and rectum.

- Treatment planning:
  - Dose can be prescribed to the vaginal surface or at a depth (typically 0.5 cm from the surface).
- Dose:
  - HDR-Boost after pelvic EBRT: 6 Gy × 2 (at 0.5 cm from surface) may be used 3 or more days apart.
  - HDR alone: 10.5 Gy × 3 (at surface) weekly. Alternative: 7 Gy × 3 (at 0.5 cm depth) weekly.

Definitive RT

- General principles:
  - EBRT to whole pelvis, as per "General Principles."
  - Brachytherapy can be used alone with small tumor (eg, <2 cm) and no demonstrable evidence of myometrial invasion (Figure 9.2).
- Localization, immobilization, and simulation:
  - Magnetic resonance imaging (MRI) should be used to evaluate the depth of tumor invasion, location, and size.
  - Variety of applicators may be used, including double tandem (Rotte "Y" Applicator), tandem plus cylinders, or Heyman capsules.
    - Dorsal lithotomy position.
    - Bladder catheter with balloon is placed.
      - CT simulation in treatment position may be used for volumetric planning.
- Target volumes and organs of interest definition:
  - For 3D planning, the GTV and CTV are the uterus.
  - Include the sigmoid colon, rectum, and bladder.

FIGURE 9.2 An 81-year-old medically inoperable woman with endometrial intraepithelial carcinoma treated with HDR brachytherapy with double tandem implant, 7.5 Gy × 5 fx. Brachytherapy plan for definitive treatment of endometrial cancer, coronal (a) and sagittal (b) views.

■ Treatment planning:
  ■ For 2D planning, specify dose at 2 cm caudally from the fundus (at midline) and 2 cm laterally.
  ■ For 3D planning (recommended), contour and prescribe to the volume of the uterus.
■ Dose:
  ■ HDR alone: 7 to 7.5 Gy × 5 fx or 6 Gy x 6 fx.
  ■ HDR and Pelvic EBRT: 6 Gy × 5 fx after EBRT, treating twice weekly.
    • There is no current standard dose or fractionation scheme; additional regimens can be found per American Brachytherapy Society guidelines (1).

CERVICAL CANCER

Indications

■ Definitive: EBRT with brachytherapy
■ Postoperative: EBRT +/- brachytherapy

External Beam Radiation in the Adjuvant or Definitive Setting

■ Localization, immobilization, and simulation:
    • Refer to the "General Principles" section for full details of WPRT
■ Target volumes and organs of interest definition:
  ■ 3D planning recommended for full nodal coverage.
  ■ Refer to "General Principles" for normal structures.
  ■ Delineate the GTV (if applicable) and CTV, including the cervix and full extent of tumor, uterus, paracervical, parametrial, and uterosacral ligaments as well as regional nodes.
    • If the distal third of the vagina is involved, inguinal nodes must be covered, with the inferior border as the vaginal introitus.
    • If the posterior vaginal wall is involved, cover the perirectal lymph nodes.
    • If the common iliac nodes are positive, raise the superior border for a 4 cm margin on known nodes. Also consider treating the PA nodes if common iliac nodes are involved.
  ■ PTV: per "General Principles."
■ Treatment planning:
  ■ Conventional techniques: either two (AP/PA) or four (AP, PA, right lateral, and left lateral) photon fields.
  ■ Four-field pelvis borders: will include GTV and CTV as defined by planning CT.

- AP/PA: superiorly cover L4-L5, 4 cm margin inferiorly/bottom of the obturator foramen to include the pelvic floor, 2 cm lateral to the bony pelvis.
- Lateral: per "General Principles"; ensure posterior coverage of at least 1.5 cm behind anterior surface of sacrum.
- For extended field, include 2 cm margin around uninvolved nodes.
  - Special considerations:
    - AP/PA fields should be used for thin patients or for uterosacral ligament involvement. Consider midline block to avoid excess dose adjacent to the implant and to deliver a higher dose to potential tumor-bearing regions outside the implant, placed at 40 Gy.
    - For stage IIB or IIIB or lymph node–positive disease, consider a boost to the parametria of an additional 5.4-9 Gy depending on response.
- Dose
  - WPRT: 45 to 50 Gy/1.8 to 2 Gy/fx.

Brachytherapy—Definitive

- General principles
  - Brachytherapy alone can be given for stage IA1 cervical cancer.
  - LDR or HDR can be used with comparable outcomes.
    - Advantages of HDR: no anesthesia, outpatient procedure, inverse treatment planning can be used to optimize source dwell positions and dwell times.
    - Disadvantages of HDR: larger fractions compared with LDR, so implant geometry must be optimal.
  - HDR with EBRT:
    - Generally begins during EBRT week 4, provided appropriate tumor reduction or immediately after EBRT.
    - At least 1 insertion per week is performed, with no EBRT or chemotherapy administered on the day of insertion.
    - If majority of EBRT has been given, then two insertions per week are performed (separated by 72 hours) to complete all therapy with an overall treatment time of less than 8 weeks.
    - Applicators include tandem and ring, tandem and ovoids, or tandem and split ring.
- Localization, immobilization, and simulation
  - Intracavitary HDR implant: tandem and ovoids/ring per "General Principles."
- Target volumes and organs of interest definition
  - Point A: in the plane of the tandem, 2 cm superior and 2 cm lateral to the external os, where the uterine artery and ureter cross.

- Point B: 5 cm lateral to the midline at the level of point A, representing the obturator LN. Point B receives approximately one-third to one-quarter of the dose to point A.
- Bladder point: posterior surface of the Foley balloon on lateral *x*-ray and center of the balloon on the AP film. Foley balloon is filled with 7 cm³ radiopaque contrast and pulled down against urethra.
- Rectal point: 5 mm behind posterior vaginal wall at midvaginal source.
- Vaginal point: lateral edge of ovoid/ring on AP film and mid-ovoid/ring on lateral film.
- If 3D planning is used, define GTV, high-risk CTV, intermediate-risk CTV, and contour normal tissues including the bladder, rectum, sigmoid colon, and vagina (see Figure 9.3).
  - The Groupe Européen de Curiethérapie and European Society for Therapeutic Radiology and Oncology (GEC-ESTRO) working group guidelines (4) recommend delineation of gross tumor volume at diagnosis (GTV_D). This includes macroscopic tumor extension at diagnosis detected by clinical examination and T2-weighted MRI. Following EBRT but prior to each brachytherapy fraction, a GTV_B is defined based on clinical examination and the T2-weighted MRI. If patients are treated with brachytherapy alone $GTV_B = GTV_D$. Next, a high-risk CTV for brachytherapy ($HR\text{-}CTV_B$) is defined and this will include the GTV_B, the whole cervix, and presumed extra-cervical tumor extension at the time of brachytherapy. In advanced disease the presumed tumor extension is delineated, taking into account the GTV_D and residual grey zones seen on MRI at the time of brachytherapy. The final incremental volume is the intermediate-risk CTV ($IR\text{-}CTV_B$); this encompasses the $HR\text{-}CTV_B$ with a safety margin of 5 to 15 mm. These margins are confined by anatomical boundaries (eg, bladder/rectal wall) if at diagnosis they were not violated by the tumor. Finally, in image-guided brachytherapy it is assumed that the PTV = $IR\text{-}CTV_B$ (2).

FIGURE 9.3 T2-weighted sagittal MRI scan of a 45-year-old patient with T2aN0M0 moderately differentiated squamous cell carcinoma of the cervix. HR-CTV delineated in orange, IR-CTV in pink, isometrically grown but restricted by uninvolved anatomical boundaries.

FIGURE 9.4 A 43-year-old woman with adenocarcinoma of the cervix, stage IB2, treated with EBRT 45 Gy with concurrent cisplatin, followed by a brachytherapy boost with a tandem and split ring to total dose of 30 Gy prescribed to point A, at 6 Gy/ fx × 5. Brachytherapy plan for cervical cancer: coronal view.

- Treatment planning
  - Classically, the dose has been prescribed to point A.
  - 3D planning and inverse treatment planning, with resultant optimization of dwell positions and times, are increasingly used to improve target coverage while minimizing dose to normal tissues (Figure 9.4).
- Dose
  - Treat point A to 80 to 85 Gy for early stage and 85 to 90 Gy for advanced stage disease.
  - The pelvic sidewall dose should be 50 to 55 Gy for early and 55 to 65 Gy for advanced-stage disease.
  - Limit bladder and rectal doses below 75 and 70 Gy LDR-equivalent doses.
  - For HDR, limit bladder and rectal dose to 65% to 70% of the prescription dose.
  - Limit upper vagina to 140 Gy and lower vagina to 90 Gy.
    - Dose specification to point A alone is insufficient. The International Commission on Radiation Units & Measurements recommends reporting dose information with technique description, reference volume, dimensions of reference volume, bladder point dose, rectal point dose, pelvic wall point dose, and lymphatic trapezoid dose.
- Special considerations
  - Indications for interstitial implant: bulky cervical cancer (vaginal or parametrial), bulky or vaginal recurrence, or cervical cancer that did not regress during EBRT.

VULVAR CANCER

Indications

- Neo-adjuvant chemoradiation for locally advanced lesions.
- Adjuvant RT to the primary site: for positive margins, positive lymph nodes, angiolymphatic invasion, or deep invasion (generally >10 mm).

■ Adjuvant RT to lymph nodes at risk: for clinically positive lymph nodes, two or more pathologically positive lymph nodes, or extracapsular extension.

■ Definitive radiation: for nonsurgical candidates.

■ Brachytherapy: as a boost for bulky disease.

External Beam Radiation Therapy

■ Localization, immobilization, and simulation:
  ■ Per "General Principles."
  ■ Special considerations:
    • Patient position: supine, frog leg position, or legs apart.
    • Wire lymph nodes, vulva, anus, and incision.
  ■ Bolus groins and vulva as needed.
■ Target volumes and organs of interest definition
  ■ Conventional field borders for 2D planning.
    • Superior: mid-SI joint (pelvic LN−) or L5/S1 (pelvic LN+)
    • Lateral:
      • AP field: include anteroinferior iliac spine (ie, medial two-thirds of inguinal ligament), or further if clips suggest more lateral involvement. No need to cover the entire scar if well beyond area at risk.
      • PA field: 2 cm beyond the bony pelvis.
    • Inferior: include the vulva, perineal skin, and medial inguinofemoral nodes; generally 2 to 3 cm below the lesser trochanter.
    • In select cases, a midline block may be added to reduce the dose to the distal urethra, vagina, anorectum, and residual vulva.
  ■ 3D planning is recommended.
  ■ If treating the primary site, contour the vulvar scar with a margin. May be included with pelvic field or en face.
  ■ If treating lymph nodes, contour the unilateral or bilateral groin nodes. Include caudal external iliac nodes if pelvic nodes are negative, or up to common iliac nodes if pelvic nodes are positive (Figure 9.5).

Treatment Planning

■ 6 MV or higher photons.
■ Variety of field arrangements can be used.
  ■ Wide AP field and narrow PA field with partial transmission block placed in the central portion of the AP field.
  ■ Match AP/PA fields to include the primary and the pelvic nodes and treat the groins through separate anterior electron fields.
  ■ IMRT is increasingly used.

FIGURE 9.5 IMRT plan for a 65-year-old woman with recurrent well-differentiated squamous cell carcinoma of the vulva status post (s/p) multiple resections, presenting with recurrence in left labia and bilateral inguinal lymph nodes. (a) Digitally reconstructed radiograph (DRR) with superimposed nodal (green) and primary (red) CTV; (b) axial and (c) coronal views with CTV delineated in red. Plan consisted of WPRT-45 Gy/1.8 Gy/fx with IMRT, with a concomitant perineal boost of 15 Gy/1.5 Gy/fx twice daily with 18 MeV electrons.

- ■ To supplement vulva for gross disease, use an en face field.
- ■ To supplement lymph nodes while respecting the femoral head tolerance, consider supplemental electrons, half-beam oblique photon fields, or IMRT.
- ■ Dose:
  - ■ Residual microscopic disease: 45 to 56 Gy/1.8 to 2 Gy/fx for adjuvant therapy.
  - ■ Residual gross disease or definitive therapy: 54 to 64 Gy at standard fractionation (up to 72 Gy without chemotherapy).

VAGINAL CANCER

Indications

- ■ For stage I patients: consider brachytherapy alone.
- ■ All other stages require a combination of EBRT and brachytherapy.
- ■ Radiation therapy is the primary treatment approach for stage II or greater disease.

External Beam Radiation Therapy

- Localization, immobilization, and simulation
  - Per "General Principles."
  - Special considerations:
    - Tumor and introital markers.
    - Bolus inguinal nodes if needed.
- Target volumes and organs of interest definition
  - Extend pelvic field border inferiorly to cover the entire vagina and 3 cm below the lowest extent of the disease.
  - If distal one-third involvement, lateral borders should include the inguinofemoral nodes.
    - Superolateral border: anterior superior iliac spine.
    - Lateral: greater trochanter.
    - Inferior: inguinal crease or 2.5 cm below the ischium.
  - Three-dimensional planning is recommended for full nodal coverage.
  - In select cases, a midline block may be added after 20 Gy to decrease dose to the bladder and rectum when brachytherapy is planned after EBRT.
- Treatment planning
  - AP/PA or 4-field.
  - 6 MV photons or higher are generally used.

Dose

- For WPRT alone, 45 to 50 Gy/1.8 to 2 Gy/fx.
- If brachytherapy is planned, treat WPRT to 45 Gy.

Brachytherapy

- General Principles
  - Use intracavitary HDR general principles for lesions less than 0.5 cm in depth. Please refer to "General Principles" for full details of intracavitary brachytherapy.
  - Use interstitial brachytherapy for lesions more than 0.5 cm in depth.
- Localization, immobilization, and simulation
  - Per "General Principles."
- Target volumes:
  - CT scan is performed for treatment planning.
  - For intracavitary brachytherapy, use the largest possible vaginal cylinder to improve the ratio of mucosa to tumor dose.
  - For interstitial implants, the depth of the tumor should be delineated to adequately cover the gross disease.

- Treatment planning
  - 3D planning and inverse treatment planning, with resultant optimization of dwell positions and times, are increasingly used to improve target coverage while minimizing dose to normal tissues.
- Dose/fractionation
  - Cylinder
    - HDR doses of 5 to 7 Gy prescribed to a depth of 0.5 cm into the entire vaginal mucosa are delivered once or twice per week, for total dose of 21 to 25 Gy delivered to the entire vaginal length.
    - An additional 21 to 25 Gy is delivered to the tumor volume using a custom-shielded vaginal cylinder, in fractions of 5 to 7 Gy prescribed to a depth of 0.5 cm.
  - Interstitial
    - Total tumor volume doses of 75 to 80 Gy from combined EBRT and brachytherapy implant.

REFERENCES

1. Nag S, Erickson B, Parikh S, et al. The American Brachytherapy Society recommendations for high-dose-rate brachytherapy for carcinoma of the endometrium. *Int J Radiat Oncol Biol Phys*. 2000;48(3):779–790.

2. Haie-Meder C, Potter R, Van Limbergen E, et al. Recommendations from Gynaecological (GYN) GEC-ESTRO Working Group (I): concepts and terms in 3D image based 3D treatment planning in cervix cancer brachytherapy with emphasis on MRI assessment of GTV and CTV. *Radiother Oncol*. 2005;74(3):235–245.

3. www.rtog.org/ClinicalTrials/ProtocolTable/StudyDetails.aspx?study=0418 (accessed October 4, 2013).

4. Potter R, Haie-Meder C, Van Limbergen E, et al. Recommendations from Gynaecological (GYN) GEC ESTRO working group (II): concepts and terms in 3D image-based treatment planning in cervix cancer brachytherapy-3D dose volume parameters and aspects of 3D image-based anatomy, radiation physics, radiobiology. *Radiother Oncol*. 2006;78:67–77

10 Lymphoma and Myeloma Radiotherapy

Jeffrey A. Kittel and Roger M. Macklis

GENERAL PRINCIPLES

- Lymphomas represent a heterogeneous group of disease entities, which make the treatment planning details largely case-specific.
- Dose prescription and target volumes will be determined by the specific disease entity.
- Lymphoma patients are ideally seen, reviewed, and examined by the treating radiation oncologist before chemotherapy to fully appreciate the initial extent of the disease.

Treatment Fields

- Field design for both Hodgkin and non-Hodgkin lymphoma (HL and NHL, respectively) follows the same general principles.
- Field boundaries and target delineation are areas of ongoing controversy, but current practice is favoring decreasing sizes of fields where possible.
- The main approaches to lymph node coverage are the following, in order of decreasing field size (for detailed descriptions, see "Target Volumes and Organs of Interest Definition"):
  - Total lymphoid irradiation (TLI): includes both mantle and inverted Y extended fields.
    - Currently rarely used.
  - Subtotal lymphoid irradiation (STLI): includes mantle and para-aortic fields, excluding pelvic LN.
  - Extended field RT (EFRT), aka "Classic fields:"
    - Mantle field: Includes all major lymph nodes above the diaphragm.
    - "Inverted Y" (aka, subdiaphragmatic field): includes para-aortic and pelvic LN plus spleen.
  - Regional field and involved field RT (IFRT):
    - Treat only portions of the classic fields.
      - Involved nodal field and first echelon uninvolved lymph node basins (regional field).
      - Involved nodal field only (IFRT).
    - Extranodal sites include entire involved organ.
  - Involved site RT (ISRT):
    - Treats the site of the originally involved nodes, possible subclinical involvement, and any extranodal extension using clinical judgment in combination with the best available pre- and posttreatment imaging to adapt fields to sites at risk after therapy.
    - Newly adopted as the standard for HL and NHL by the National Comprehensive Cancer Network (NCCN)
  - Involved node RT (INRT):
    - Treats only involved nodes as defined by optimal imaging, including pretreatment FDG-PET scans, to adapt fields to sites at risk after therapy.
    - Considered a special case of ISRT.

Localization, Immobilization, and Simulation

- Volumetric treatment planning (CT simulation on a flat surface) for definition of GTV, CTV, and PTV.
- Positioning:
  - Supine with the neck extended and arms above the head draws axillary LN farther from the chest wall, permitting more generous lung shielding.

■ Children: consider arms akimbo.
  ● Permits humeral head shielding, minimizing tissue folds in supra-clavicular and low neck regions.
■ Immobilization:
  ■ Numerous systems (eg, vacuum-lock bag and thermoplastic mold) are commercially available to position the arms above the head in a repro-ducible, patient-friendly manner. When treating disease in the head-and-neck region, a thermoplastic mask should be used.

Target Definition

■ Palpable lymph nodes should be wired for visualization at the time of simulation.
■ Reference all prechemotherapy and postchemotherapy CT scans
■ Reference prechemotherapy PET-CT
  ■ If RT planning preceedes PET, PET scan should be performed in the treatment position with immobilization
■ Remission status after chemotherapy should be determined for each ini-tially involved lymph node using CT or PET scans per the criteria detailed in Table 10.1.

Target Volumes and Organs of Interest Definition

■ "Classic" lymphoma fields provide the foundation for understanding how contemporary external beam radiotherapy fields have evolved.
■ Required to understand long-term results for disease outcome and toxicity data.
■ Mantle field (see Figure 10.1)
  ■ Superior border includes the inferior portion of the mandible and mas-toid tip. Inferior border should be near the insertion of the diaphragm (T10-11).
  ■ Laterally, the field should include the axilla, splitting the humeral head.
  ■ Lung blocks conform to the mediastinal contour, no more than 0.5 cm margins around the involved LN. Include the pulmonary hilar LN. The superior extent of lung blocks is drawn to expose the infraclavicular region (lymphatic channels here communicate with the axillary and supraclavicular LN regions). Therefore, lung blocks should begin at the 3rd rib and extend down laterally to the 6th rib.
  ■ Laryngeal block may be placed over the inferior half of thyroid cartilage and cricoid cartilage from the start or at 20 Gy (as long as not blocking disease). A posterior cervical cord block (5 HVL) may be considered if the total dose to the cord is calculated to be high (usually for doses >40 Gy, not needed for doses up to 36 Gy).

TABLE 10.1 Response Criteria for Lymphoma

	IWC CT Criteria	PET Criteria
CR	Complete disappearance of clinically and/or radiologically detectable disease	–CR by IWC with a completely negative PET –CRu, PR, or SD by IWC with a completely negative PET and a negative BMB if positive prior to therapy –PD by IWC with a completely negative PET and CT abnormalities (new lesion, increasing size of previous lesion), 1.5 cm (1.0 cm in the lungs), and negative BMB if positive prior to therapy
CRu	At least a 75% decrease in tumor size	–CRu by IWC with a completely negative PET but with an indeterminate BMB
PR	At least a 50% decrease in tumor size	–CR, CRu, or PR by IWC with a positive PET at the site of a previously involved node/nodal mass –CR, CRu, PR, or SD by IWC with a positive PET outside the site of a previously involved node/nodal mass –SD by IWC with a positive PET at the site of a previously involved node/nodal mass that regressed to <1.5 cm if previously >1.5 cm, or <1 cm if previously 1.1–1.5 cm
Failure	<50% decrease or any increase in tumor size	–PD by IWC with a positive PET finding corresponding to the CT abnormality (new lesion, increasing size of previous lesion) –PD by IWC with a negative PET and a CT abnormality (new lesion, increasing size of previous lesion) of <1.5 cm (<1.0 cm in the lungs)

Abbreviations: BMB, bone marrow biopsy; CR, complete remission; CRu, unconfirmed complete remission; CT, computed tomography; IWC, International Workshop Criteria; PD, progressive disease; PR, partial response; SD, stable disease.

Source: Adapted from Refs. 1 and 2.

FIGURE 10.1 AP mantle field without (a) and with (b) heart block. Carina is delineated in green for reference.

- For patients with extension to the pericardium or significant inferior extension of the mediastinal mass, treat the entire cardiac silhouette to 15 Gy, then place a block over the left ventricular apex. A subcarinal block (5 cm below the carina) is placed after 30 Gy to further shield the heart.
- Inverted-Y field (see Figure 10.2)
  - Superior border is matched with the mantle with appropriate gap calculation (overlap at 10 cm depth may be used; gap is on the order of 2–3 cm).
  - Right lateral extent to the transverse process or to encompass the involved LN with 1 cm margin and left lateral extent to the rib cage to include the entire spleen (including surgical clips and 2 cm margin to account for respiratory motion).
  - Definition of the iliac nodes is best accomplished by lymphangiography or CT, with a 0.5 cm margin around lymphatic bed.
  - Inferior border for the para-aortic portion is at L4-L5, after which the pelvic field extends laterally 1.5 to 2 cm past the widest point of the bony pelvis and inferiorly to at least the lesser trochanters.
  - Borders may be modified if there is disease that extends past these landmarks or if radiographic studies are used to more accurately delineate nodal anatomy.
  - In males, a midline block is placed, and testicular shielding is used to reduce the dose to 0.75% to 3% of the prescription dose, which is predominately from internal scatter.
  - In females, the inferior border should not be any lower than the superior level of the sacroiliac joints unless an oophoropexy has been performed, to limit the scatter dose of radiation to the ovaries. A 10-HVL block is placed to shield transposed ovaries after oophoropexy.

FIGURE 10.2 Inverted-Y field. Para-aortic lymph nodes are delineated in green; pelvic lymph nodes, in red; spleen, in blue; and kidneys, in light blue.

- Regional field
  - Involved field (per Table 10.2) plus at least one adjacent clinically uninvolved region
  - Extranodal disease: Treat involved organ or area and draining lymph node region.
- IFRT Special considerations for field choice include:
  - Cervical/SCV disease: Treat bilateral fields if bilateral nodes are involved.
  - Mediastinal disease: If one cervical chain involved, include unilateral cervical field blocking contralateral neck as described in Table 10.2. If both cervical regions involved, treat mantle field without axilla.
  - Extranodal disease: Treat either whole involved organ or affected portion.
- ISRT
  - Prechemotherapy GTV (pre-GTV) is defined by clinical judgment of involved areas based on best available imaging.
  - Postchemotherapy CT or PET/CT is used to delineate postchemotherapy GTV (post-GTV, if applicable).
  - Postchemotherapy CTV = pre-GTV + post-GTV + margin
    - If possible, fuse preop imaging, including pre-GTV with simulation CT, then contour post-GTV (if applicable).
    - Expand pre-GTV + post-GTV to accommodate uncertainty associated with suboptimal prechemotherapy imaging (eg, lack of PET, different patient positioning, substantial time between imaging and start of chemo), often by approximately 1 to 2 cm depending on degree of uncertainty (3).
    - Exclude normal structures uninvolved by lymphoma (eg, vessels, muscle, bone, lungs, kidneys, etc.) using clinical judgment.

- Adapt to anatomical changes between prechemotherapy and post-chemotherapy scans.
  - In the mediastinum, the superior-inferior dimension of the CTV should remain the same as that of the prechemotherapy volume. The lateral boundaries of the CTV should not exceed the normal mediastinum or lymph node remnants.
  - If no prechemotherapy imaging is available, use clinical judgment and all available information to determine post-CTV.
  - As a rule, post-CTV should be larger than for INRT (see below).
  - If the initially involved lymph nodes are more than 5 cm apart, may need to define separate CTVs.
- Further CTV modification according to clinical response to chemo (Table 10.1):
  - Complete remission (CR) or CRu: In case of a CRu, the lymph node remnant should be included in the CTV.
  - Partial response (PR): Two PTVs should be outlined: PTV1 is the expansion on the pre-GTVPET + pre-GTVCT + post-GTV and PTV2 is the expansion on the post-GTV alone.
- ITV = CTV + margin to accommodate tumor motion.
  - Techniques include 4D-CT, fluoroscopy, or differential expansion (eg, 1.5–2 cm in superior-inferior directions).
- PTV = CTV (or ITV) + margin to accommodate setup uncertainty
  - Institution or clinician-dependent, depending on immobilization, body site, etc. In mediastinum, 0.5 to 1 cm is often considered sufficient.
- INRT: Considered a special case of ISRT (8).
  - Prechemotherapy CT is used to delineate the pre-GTVCT.
  - Prechemotherapy PET is used to delineate the pre-GTVPET.
  - Prechemotherapy PET/CT, pre-GTVCT, and pre-GTVPET are fused to postchemotherapy simulation CT.
  - Postchemotherapy CT or PET/CT is fused to postchemotherapy simulation CT and is used to delineate post-GTV (if present).
  - Postchemotherapy CTV = pre-GTVCT + pre-GTVPET + post-GTV.
    - No expansion from GTV to CTV.
    - Modify postchemotherapy CTV according to normal tissue boundaries and clinical response to chemo, as described in ISRT (see above).
  - ITV = CTV + margin to accommodate tumor motion, as described in ISRT (see above).
  - PTV = CTV (or ITV) + margin to accommodate setup uncertainty, as described in ISRT (see above).
- Normal anatomy to be routinely identified.
  - Lungs (right and left done separately, then combined as a composite lung volume).

TABLE 10.2 Borders of Involved Fields

Nodal Region	Superior	Inferior
Cervical/SCV (see Figure 10.3)	1–2 cm above the lower tip of the mastoid process and midpoint through the chin	2 cm below the clavicle
Mediastinum/ hilum (see Figure 10.4)	C5-C6 interspace – top of larynx if SCV involved, bottom of larynx if SCV not involved	5 cm below the carina, or 2 cm below prechemother- apy GTV
Axillary (see Figure 10.5)	C5-C6 interspace	Lower tip of the scapula, or 2 cm below lowest axillary node
Para-aortic/spleen (see Figure 10.2, green, area represents PA field)	Top of T11, or at least 2 cm above prechemotherapy GTV	Bottom of L4, or at least 2 cm below preche- motherapy GTV
Inguinal/femoral/ external iliac (see Figure 10.2, red area represents inguinal field)	Mid-SI joint	5 cm below lesser trochanter to include femoral LNs

Abbreviations: GTV, gross tumor volume; ICV, infraclavicular; PA, posteroanterior; SI, sacroiliac; SCV, supraclavicular.

Lateral	Medial	Notes
Include medial ⅔ of the clavicle	SCV uninvolved Ipsilateral transverse process. If medial nodes, include entire vertebral body SCV involved Contralateral transverse process	Head hyperextended, arms at the side. Laryngeal block, add at 19.8 Gy if involved nodes. Posterior cervical cord block if dose >40 Gy. Posterior mouth block if supine. If stage I, block larynx and vertebral bodies above larynx.
Postchemo-therapy GTV + 1.5 cm margin	N/A	Include B/L hila + 1 cm if uninvolved and 1.5 cm if involved. Arms up if axillary nodes are involved; otherwise, arms akimbo or at the sides.
Flash axilla	Ipsilateral transverse process. Include vertebral bodies if SCV involved	Arms up. Includes SCV and ICV nodal regions.
Edge of transverse process, or at least 2 cm from postchemotherapy GTV	N/A	Arms at sides. Include porta hepatis if involved. Contour kidneys for blocks. Consider renal perfusion study.
Greater trochanter, or at least 2 cm from prechemotherapy GTV. If negative split femur.	Medial border of obturator foramen, or at least 2 cm from prechemotherapy GTV	If common iliac nodes involved, extend to L4-L5 interspace, at least 2 cm above prechemotherapy GTV. Consider slight frog leg. Double shield testicles with clamshell and cerrobend.

FIGURE 10.3 Cervical lymph node fields: unilateral (a) and bilateral (b). Nodal disease is indicated in yellow, and carina is in green for reference.

■ Heart: from its base (Radiation Therapy Oncology Group (RTOG) definition: beginning at the CT slice where the ascending aorta originates and encompassing the great vessels) to the apex.
■ Kidneys: may require blocking to limit dose.
■ Spinal cord: should be contoured on each CT slice.
■ Liver: as needed, based on tumor location and field size.

Treatment Planning

Therapy

■ If a conventional treatment is used with AP/PA fields, the size of the field should be at least 5 × 5 cm.
  Consider AP/PA with differential weighting.
  ■ While 2-dimensional treatment planning was used traditionally, 3D planning has become standard.

FIGURE 10.4 Mediastinal field. Disease is delineated in yellow, and carina is in green for reference.

FIGURE 10.5 Axillary field. Disease is delineated in yellow, and carina is in green for reference.

- 2D techniques have been adapted to 3D treatment planning to cover the same areas at risk while restricting the dose to the normal tissues. IMRT is generally avoided due to concerns over higher integral dose, especially in young patients.

Critical Structures

- Doses to critical structures are usually well within tolerance for the majority of the dose prescriptions used for the treatment of lymphoma, except potentially for lung, liver, and heart.
- Lungs, spinal cord, heart, larynx, and kidneys should be blocked as described in "Target Volumes and Organs of Interest Definition."

Technical Factors

Beam energies
- Photon energies: 6 MV to 10 MV

Beam shaping
- Multileaf collimation or individually shaped (5 HVL) custom blocks for normal tissue protection outside the target volume are used.

Heterogeneity Corrections

- Most dose prescriptions for chest tumors have typically been based on an assumption of homogenous tissue densities. Recently, there has been a move in radiation therapy practice to distinguish the heterogeneous nature to more accurately predict dose, dose deposition, normal tissues toxicities, and outcomes. Therefore, heterogeneity corrections are now recommended in general treatment planning.

HODGKIN LYMPHOMA

General Principles

- Stage at presentation determines treatment selection (9).
- Curative EBRT may be considered for patients with early-stage disease (IA or IIA) as a function of patient and disease variables.
  - Most patients with early-stage disease are now treated with abbreviated chemotherapy and IFRT rather than with radiation therapy alone.
  - Patients with early-stage nodular lymphocyte predominant HL may be treated with radiation therapy alone.
  - Patients of any stage with bulky disease or incomplete response are usually treated with combined chemotherapy and EBRT.

Technical Factors

Field arrangement
- If treating with radiotherapy alone, wide fields are preferred to cover subclinical LN (see "Target Volumes and Organs of Interest Definition" in "General Principles," above).
- If treating with AP/PA fields, consider differential weighting to optimize dose distribution based on the burden of disease.

Dose/Fractionation

- There is some controversy with respect to dose in HL.
- Current standard doses range from 30 to 40 Gy with conventional fractionation (1.8–2 Gy/fx), with consideration given to an additional 4 to 10 Gy boost to sites of residual disease or for unfavorable risk groups.
- General dose guidelines.
  - Definitive radiation.
    - Clinically uninvolved sites, 30 Gy; boost involved sites to 36 to 40 Gy.
  - Adjuvant radiation.
    - Stage I to II, non-bulky:
      - CR: 20 to 30 Gy after ABVD, 30 Gy after Stanford V.
      - PR: 30 to 35 Gy.
    - Bulky disease (all stages):
      - CR: 30 to 36 Gy after ABVD, 36 Gy with Stanford V.
      - PR: 36 to 40 Gy.
    - With abbreviated chemotherapy for bulky or advanced stage: 36 Gy.
    - Pediatric patients: 21 to 24 Gy.

NON-HODGKIN LYMPHOMA

General Principles

- Non-Hodgkin lymphoma is composed of more than 40 distinct clinical/histological entities (10).
- This section focuses on the most common entities: diffuse large B-cell, mantle, follicular, and extranodal marginal zone large B-cell (MALT) lymphomas.

Indolent Lymphomas

Low-grade follicular lymphoma
- One-third of cases are early-stage, and IFRT is used for cure.
- Doses used ranged from 25 to 40 Gy with conventional fractionation (1.8–2 Gy/fx).

Extranodal marginal zone large B-cell lymphoma
- Disease of extranodal sites (ie, stomach, salivary glands, Waldeyer ring, thyroid, eye, intestine, etc.) (11)
- Gastric MALTs:
  - RT indicated in the setting of no response or progression after standard management ("triple therapy:" proton pump inhibitor (PPI), clarithromycin, and amoxicillin [or metronidazole]).
  - IFRT to stomach, perigastric, and celiac LNs to 30 to 35 Gy.
  - Simulation and planning approach.
    - Oral contrast given at simulation.
    - Entire stomach (GTV) and target nodal groups are contoured.
    - Stomach contour expanded by several centimeters (~3–5) to encompass target lymph nodes.
    - Patient instructed to have empty stomach for simulation and daily for treatment.
    - AP/PA fields were traditionally used.
    - 3D conformal treatment with complex field arrangements now favored to spare ipsilateral kidney.
- Nongastric MALTs are usually treated with IFRT to 24 to 36 Gy.
- Orbital MALT: May be treated with 25 to 30 Gy. Options for field arrangement include IMRT, opposed laterals (D-shaped if attempting to spare lenses), or anterior electrons with lens shielding.

Relapsed or refractory low-grade lymphomas
- Can be treated palliatively with doses as low as 4 Gy in 2 fx with excellent response and control rates.

Diffuse large B-cell lymphoma

■ Dose/Fractionation largely determined by stage, response to chemo, risk factors, number of cycles of chemotherapy (10,11).

   ■ Early stage: after chemotherapy, IFRT to 30-36 Gy for CR, 40 to 50 Gy for PR.

   ■ Advanced stage: may consider RT after chemo for bulky or residual disease, but this is controversial.

Mantle cell lymphoma

■ Because this often presents as stage IV, EBRT is indicated only in rare cases, such as combined chemoradiation for stages I to II, especially for bulky disease.

■ Doses range from 15 to 30 Gy.

RADIOIMMUNOTHERAPY

General Principles

■ Two radioimmunopharmaceutical agents are Food and Drug Administration (FDA)-approved for the treatment of relapsed or refractory low-grade, follicular, or transformed B-cell NHL, including patients with rituximab refractory follicular NHL; Bexxar is also indicated for transformed CD20+ NHL.

   ■ Zevalin (Spectrum Pharmaceuticals, Irvine, California)—ibritumomab tiuxetan: Yttrium-90 labeled IgG k murine monoclonal anti-CD20 antibody. A separate isotope, Indium-111, is used for imaging, e-capture decay, 2.8-day half-life.

   ■ Bexxar (GlaxoSmithKline, Brentford, Middlesex, United Kingdom)—tositumomab: Iodine-131 labeled IgG murine anti-CD20 antibody. Dose is based on individual patient pharmacokinetics due to variable excretion.

   ■ Table 10.3 summarizes the main characteristics of both agents.

■ Contraindications.

   ■ Greater than 25% marrow involvement.

   ■ Impaired bone marrow reserve:

      ● Prior external beam RT to greater than 25% of the marrow.

      ● Platelet count less than 100,000.

      ● Neutrophil count less than 1,500.

   ■ Altered biodistribution based on pretreatment imaging.

   ■ Human antimouse antibodies for Bexxar.

TABLE 10.3 Characteristics of Commonly Used Radioimmunotherapy Agents

Table LJ-Lymph-4	Zevalin	Bexxar
Antibody		
Predose (cold)	Chimeric (rituximab, RTX)	Murine (tositumomab, TST)
Radiolabeled	Murine IgG1	Murine IgG2
Total dose	250 mg/m^2 × 2	485 mg/m^2 × 2
Isotope	Yttrium-90	Iodine-131
T½ physical	2.7 d	8.0 d
Maximum energy	2.3 MeV β only	0.6 MeV β + 364 keV γ
Mean path length	5.3 mm (~150 cell diam)	0.80 mm
Nontumor uptake	Bone	Thyroid
Dosing		
Platelets >150,000	0.4 mCi/kg	75 cGy whole body dose
Platelets 100–150,000	0.3 mCi/kg (max 32 mCi)	65 cGy whole body dose
Estimated whole body dose	60 cGy	75/65 cGy
Mean tumor dose	1,700 cGy	895 cGy

Administration

- There are several steps to successful radioimmunotherapy requiring multidisciplinary coordination. Table 10.4 summarizes the treatment steps for both Zevalin and Bexxar.

MYCOSIS FUNGOIDES

General Principles

- Radiation therapy is indicated in the definitive management of localized disease and in symptomatic palliation of disseminated cutaneous, nodal, and/or visceral lesions.
  - Stage IA mycosis fungoides is most often treated locally with superficial electron beam radiation therapy.
  - For T2 to T4 diseases, either multiple fields encompassing the main disease sites or total skin electron beam therapy (TSEBT) can be used as a primary treatment.

TABLE 10.4 Steps in Administration of Radioimmunotherapy

Day	Description	Details
0	Patient selection	Pretreatment bone marrow biopsy and imaging
0	Cold antibody RTX: Zevalin (Z) TST: Bexxar (B)	Unlabeled antibody (Ab) optimizes the radiolabeled antibody by binding to B lymphocytes and cells with Fc receptors (spleen). Thus, cold Ab blocks binding of the radiolabeled antibody to the normal organs and depletes normal B cells. It also allows deeper penetration and more homogenous distribution. Note: dose for cold Ab in Zevalin administration is 250 mg RTX compared with 375 mg/m^2 for RTX alone.
0 + 4	Trace dose	A small (5 mCi) dose of radiolabeled antibody is given to assess biodistribution and ensure that pooling does not occur. For Zevalin, Indium-111 is conjugated to ibritumomab instead of Yttrium-90, which cannot be imaged due to its pure β emission. The same antibody/isotope is used for imaging and treatment in the case of Bexxar.
1, 2 (Z) 0, 2, and 6 (B)	Imaging Third Zevalin scan on day 4 is optional	Gamma camera images are obtained by nuclear medicine. For Zevalin, these scans are used to ensure that pooling does not occur. Bexxar scans are used to calculate the clearance and therapeutic dose because elimination is less predictable than Yttrium-90. This allows for the same area under the curve for patients who have fast and slow clearance. For Zevalin, absorbed dose by the marrow is not predictive of toxicity; hence, detailed dosimetry is not required. Altered biodistribution for Z is defined as high accumulation in the lung > the heart on image 1, or lung > kidney or liver on images 2–3, kidneys > liver on posteroanterior view of day 2 or 3, uptake in normal bowel > liver on days 2 and 3.

(*continued*)

TABLE 10.4 Steps in Administration of Radioimmunotherapy (*continued*)

Day	Description	Details
7	Thyroid cytoprotection (Bexxar only)	In the case of Bexxar, as the joined antibody is broken down, free Iodine-131 floats in the blood stream, and it can be absorbed by the thyroid, resulting in hypothyroidism. Therefore, 1 day before treatment, Lugol solution/potassium iodide is started and continued for 14 days after treatment to saturate iodine uptake by the thyroid.
8	Treatment	Dosing is based on weight/platelet count for Zevalin and clearance/platelet count for Bexxar (see Table 10.3 above). Infuse over several minutes, monitoring for any infusion related reactions. Radiation safety precautions need to be observed closely.
8	Release instructions	Most (and essentially all Zevalin) patients qualify for immediate release. The γ emission of Iodine-131 requires specific instructions to the Bexxar patient to sleep in a separate bed, not take a long trip, maintain >6 ft from others, avoid contact with children and pregnant women, etc.

Localization, Immobilization, and Simulation

▪ Variable depending on the site being treated and on the type of treatment approach used.
▪ TSEBT will be discussed in a separate section.

Target Volumes and Organs of Interest Definition

▪ Stage IA mycosis fungoides.
  ▪ Disease area with a 2 to 3 cm margin, ensuring coverage to a depth of 4 mm
  ▪ A single radiation field should be used whenever possible.
  ▪ When matching fields due to size or geometric constraints, feathering of the field junctions should be done on a weekly basis to maximize dose homogeneity.
▪ Stage IB, II, and III mycosis fungoides.
  ▪ Multiple fields as defined in stage IA can be used to treat the main disease sites of more advanced disease.

■ TSEBT also used

- Target volume of stage IB and II diseases to include the epidermis and dermis.
- Target volume of stage III (cutaneous tumors) disease to include the full depth of the tumors.

Treatment Planning

Focal therapy

■ Usually, a clinical setup for en–face electron fields, superficial X-ray units, or higher-energy photons (eg, 6 MV) with bolus.

Critical Structures

■ Clinical setup and technique will always take neighboring normal structures into account at the time of simulation (eg, skin folds, eyelid, etc.), often resulting in complex clinical setups.

Technical Factors

Beam energies

■ Selection based on tumor characteristics.
■ Electron beam (6–12 MeV), superficial X-rays, or higher energy photons (eg, 6 MV) with bolus.

Beam shaping

■ Electron cutouts mounted on the corresponding cones are used for beam shaping.

Dose/Fractionation

■ Stage IA mycosis fungoides
  ■ Approximately 20 to 30 Gy in 1.8 to 2 Gy/fx.
  ■ Stage IB, II, and III mycosis fungoides:
    - When using multiple fields, the same guidelines as for stage IA apply.

Total skin electron beam therapy (TSEBT)

■ Delivered over 9 weeks, 1 Gy per day, 4 days per week, with a 1-week break after week 4, to a total dose of 36 Gy (36 treatment days).
  ■ For TSEBT, 26 Gy or greater should be prescribed to a depth of 4 mm, with a surface dose of 31 to 36 Gy (4).
  ■ A boost treatment to bulky or symptomatic areas 1 to 2 weeks prior to the delivery of TSEBT may be used.

FIGURE 10.6 Six treatment positions (left to right) used for total skin treatment: anteroposterior, right anterior oblique, left anterior oblique, posteroanterior, right posterior oblique, and left posterior oblique.

- 4 to 6 Gy in a single fraction, or 10 to 20 Gy in 5 to 10 fx, using en face electrons (energy dependent on target depth) with 1 cm margins.
- Six treatment positions ensure complete skin coverage (Figure 10.6).
- The treatment cycle consists of 3 of the 6 fields treated per day alternating over the 4 day weekly cycle.
  - The weekly schedule (only 4 treatment days) is AP/right posterior oblique/left posterior oblique on day 1 and PA/right anterior oblique/left anterior oblique on day 2, repeat for days 3 and 4.
  - This cycle is repeated 9 times.
- Each treatment position is treated with a split field to maximize dose homogeneity.
- Use nail and eye blocks to prevent overdosing these areas.

- In these treatment positions, the soles of the feet, scalp, inframammary, pannicular, perianal, buttocks/thighs, inner thighs, and perineal skin regions may be underdosed.
  - Some recommend patch treatment to the underdosed areas.

MULTIPLE MYELOMA/PLASMACYTOMA

General Principles

- EBRT only for palliation in the management of multiple myeloma
- Indications for palliation include pain related to bone or soft tissue disease, for neurological compromise, or for pathologic fracture or impending pathologic fracture after orthopedic stabilization (5).
- Radiation is usually given in a sequential fashion with relation to chemotherapy, as toxicity from concurrent treatment can be great.

Localization, Immobilization, and Simulation

- Variable depending on the site being treated. Usually, the patient is supine without any special immobilization, but proper reproducibility of setup in the target site is ensured.

Target Volumes and Organs of Interest Definition

- The radiographic lesion(s) plus a 2 cm margin. Coverage of the entire bone is not needed in long bones, except in cases where almost the entirety of the bone would get treated otherwise and whole bone treatment would allow for easier field matches in the future.
  - For vertebral lesions, the entire vertebra should be included with 1 or 2 vertebral bodies above and below.
  - Hemibody radiation was used in the past for consolidation after chemotherapy but has now fallen out of favor.

Treatment Planning

Therapy
- Conventional treatment planning is sufficient for the majority of treatments, usually with AP/PA field arrangement.
- Where there is soft tissue disease or nearby critical structures to be avoided, 3D CT-based treatment planning may be of use.

Critical Structures

- Doses used for treatment of myeloma rarely exceed normal tissue tolerance, and normal structures are not routinely delineated. For specific cases where tolerances could be exceeded, 3D treatment planning is done and structures are limited according to traditional dose constraints as explained elsewhere in this text.

Technical Factors

Beam energies
▪ Photon energies: 6 to 10 MV.

Beam shaping
▪ Multileaf collimation or individually shaped (5 HVL) custom blocks for normal tissue protection outside the target volume are used.

Dose/Fractionation

▪ The most commonly used dosing schemes for bone pain palliation are 20 to 30 Gy in 5 to 15 fx (2–4 Gy/fx). Multiple myeloma is especially radiosensitive; consider 15 to 20 Gy or single fraction (8–10 Gy).
▪ Treatment fields should be limited to spare bone marrow reserves.
▪ In the setting of spinal cord compression caused by multiple myeloma, long-course radiation (eg, 30 Gy in 10 fx) should be used (6).

SOLITARY PLASMACYTOMA OF BONE (OSSEOUS PLASMACYTOMA)

▪ Radiation therapy is the standard of care for solitary plasmacytoma of the bone, with surgery used for pathological fracture or stabilization of impending fractures and radiation given adjuvantly (7).

Immobilization and Simulation

▪ Variable depending on the site being treated. Usually, the patient is supine without any special immobilization, but proper reproducibility of setup in the target site is ensured.

Target Volumes and Organs of Interest Definition

▪ The radiographic or clinically defined lesion(s) plus a 2 to 3 cm margin
▪ For vertebral lesions, the entire vertebra should be included with 1 or 2 vertebral bodies above and below.

Treatment Planning

Therapy
▪ Conventional treatment planning is sufficient for the majority of treatments, usually with AP/PA field arrangement.

■ Where there is soft tissue disease or nearby critical structures to be avoided, 3D CT-based treatment planning may be of use.

Critical Structures

■ As a function of disease location and the dose used.

Technical Factors

Beam energies
■ Photon energies: 6 to 10 MV.

Beam shaping
■ Multileaf collimation or individually shaped (5 HVL) custom blocks for normal tissue protection outside the target volume are used.

Dose/Fractionation

■ Doses of 40 to 50 Gy/2 Gy/fx are the most frequently used regimens.

EXTRAMEDULLARY PLASMACYTOMA

■ Radiation therapy is the standard of care for extramedullary plasmacytoma.

Localization, Immobilization, and Simulation

■ Variable depending on the site being treated. Usually, the patient is supine without any special immobilization, but proper reproducibility of setup in the target site is ensured.

Target Volumes and Organs of Interest Definition

■ The radiographic or clinically defined lesion(s) plus a 2 to 3 cm margin.

Treatment Planning

Therapy
■ Conventional treatment planning is sufficient for the majority of treatments, usually with AP/PA field arrangement.
■ Where there is soft tissue disease or nearby critical structures to be avoided, 3D CT-based treatment planning may be of use.

Critical Structures

■ As a function of disease location and the dose used.

Technical Factors

Beam energies
▪ Photon energies: 6 to 10 MV.

Beam shaping
▪ Multileaf collimation or individually shaped (5 HVL) custom blocks for normal tissue protection outside the target volume are used.

Dose/Fractionation

▪ Doses of 40 to 50 Gy in 20 to 25 fx are the most frequently used regimens.
  ▪ 50 Gy recommended for bulky disease.

TOTAL BODY IRRADIATION

General Principles

▪ Used on its own, or as an adjunct to chemotherapy as part of a myeloablative regimen, to condition the host bone marrow prior to receiving a hematopoietic transplantation.
▪ There is no standard treatment technique for TBI; significant differences in dose distributions exist with different treatment methods.
▪ Techniques include:
  ▪ AP/PA with a laying patient (supine and prone) being scanned through a fixed beam.
  ▪ AP/PA with a laying patient (supine and prone) with rotating gantry head sweeping across the patient.
  ▪ Arcs, helical tomotherapy, and others.

Localization, Immobilization, and Simulation

▪ Variety of total body irradiation (TBI) techniques.
▪ Goal: to deliver low-dose rate RT (5–10 cGy/min) to a uniformity of $\pm 10\%$ to the midline at the umbilicus.
▪ To achieve a 90% or higher surface dose, a 1 to 2 cm–thick acrylic is placed 10 cm in front of the patient (known as a beam spoiler).

Opposed laterals technique
One needs to be aware of the lateral dose effect (ratio of D_{max} dose to mid-dose) due to the reduced thickness in the extremities.

▪ The patient is seated and treated with opposed lateral fields, using 10 MV photon beams and tissue compensators mounted on a tray to produce dose uniformity to within $\pm 10\%$ compared with prescription dose at midpoint at umbilicus.

- The patient's back is supported on the couch.
- Arms follow the body contour and shadow the lungs; however, using the arms to shield the lungs results in nonuniform dosimetry and compensators are recommended.

AP/PA technique
Provides better dose homogeneity and less need for tissue compensation (with the exception of lung blocks)

- The patient is in a standing position at 410 cm SAD pseudoisocentric AP/PA at the level of the umbilicus.
- 40 × 40 cm field with collimator rotated 45°.
- Harness and arm/leg rods assist in reproducibility.
- Partial transmission lung blocks are used to shield the lungs and screwed on to plastic supports close to the patient.
- Physician draws lung blocks on AP and PA films, with 1 to 1.5 cm margin around the lung border.
- Thickness of lung shielding variable: Some institutions use 1 HVL throughout the treatment course, whereas others have used a single 7-HVL block for a single fraction only. With 1 HVL and other intermediate HVL values, thermoluminescent dosimeter (TLD) is performed with and without blocks to calculate the necessary number of blocked fractions for lungs to receive ~85% of prescribed dose.

Technical Factors

Beam energies
- Photon energies: 6 to 10 MV.

Beam shaping
- Cerrobend block used for lungs as described above

Dose/Fractionation

- Dosage depends on indication and institutional protocol but may range from 4 Gy in 2 fx to 12 Gy in 6 to 8 fx.
- Testicles are boosted in male patients with leukemia, typically 4 Gy in 2 fx.

REFERENCES

1. Cheson BD, Horning SJ, Coiffer B, et al. Report of an international workshop to standardize response criteria for non-Hodgkin's lymphomas. NCI Sponsored International Working Group. *J Clin Oncol.* 1999;17:1244.

2. Juweid ME, Wiseman GA, Vose JM, et al. Response assessment of aggressive non-Hodgkin's lymphoma by integrated International Workshop Criteria and fuorine-18-fuorodeoxyglucose positron emission tomography. *J Clin Oncol.* 2005;23:4652–4661.

3. Yahalom J, Mauch P. The involved field is back: issues in delineating the radiation field in Hodgkin's disease. *Ann Oncol.* 2002;13(suppl 1):79–83.

4. Jones GW, Kacinski BM, Wilson LD, et al. Total skin electron radiation in the management of mycosis fungoides: consensus of the European Organization for Research and Treatment of Cancer (EORTC) Cutaneous Lymphoma Project Group. *J Am Acad Dermatol.* 2002;47:364–370.

5. NCCN Guidelines. Multiple Myeloma. Version 2.2013.

6. Rades D, Hoskin PJ, Stalpers LJ, et al. Short-course radiotherapy is not optimal for spinal cord compression due to myeloma. *Int J Radiat Oncol Biol Phys.* 2006;64(5):1452–1457.

7. Knobel D, Zouhair A, Tsang RW, et al. Prognostic factors in solitary plasmacytoma of the bone: a multicenter Rare Cancer Network study. *BMC Cancer.* 2006;6:118.

8. Specht L, Yahalom J, Illidge T, et al. Modern radiation therapy for Hodgkin Lymphoma: field and dose guidelines from the International Lymphoma Radiation Oncology group (ILROG). *Int J Radiation Oncol Biol Phys.* 2013;5 [Epub ahead of print].

9. NCCN Guidelines. Hodgkin's Lymphoma. Version 2.2013.

10. NCCN Guidelines. Non-Hodgkin's Lymphomas. Version 1.2013.

11. Ng A, Yahalom J. Updated roles and rules for radiation therapy of indolent and aggressive lymphomas. *ASTRO Educational Session.* 2012. www.astro.org

11   Soft Tissue Sarcoma Radiotherapy

Neil M. Woody, Kevin L. Stephans, Samuel T. Chao, and Erin S. Murphy

GENERAL PRINCIPLES

- Surgical resection is the foundation of sarcoma treatment.
- External beam radiation (EBRT) and brachytherapy techniques are used in the preoperative and postoperative settings for the extremities, trunk, and in the retroperitoneum.

Localization, Immobilization, and Simulation

- Localization
  - Spiral computed tomography (CT) with 3 mm slices spanning the target region.
  - Large bore scanner gives maximum flexibility in arranging the limb so that the contralateral extremity and trunk are out of the beam.
  - Intravenous contrast is not typically used.

- Immobilization
  - Positioning is highly dependent on the site.
  - Most patients are positioned supine; the affected extremities are positioned to maximize reproducibility and treatment angle options while minimizing exposure to adjacent structures.
  - Vacuum-locking bags and body molds aid in making positioning reproducible.
- Simulation
  - Radiopaque wires are used to mark biopsy site (preoperative) or surgical incision (postoperative).
  - Bolus should be considered over the scar in the postoperative setting.
  - Isocenter is placed at least D_{max} depth from the surface and typically in a central location within the anticipated treatment volume.

Target Volumes and Organs of Interest Definition

- Knowledge of muscle compartments and fascial planes is mandatory for appropriate treatment planning.
- Target volumes typically include gross disease, tumor bed, and surgical scar.
- Dose-limiting normal structures vary depending on site and should be delineated on planning CT if located near the target volumes.
- Surrounding normal structures are delineated for dose assessment at the time of treatment planning.
- Preoperative and postoperative diagnostic imaging studies are used to aid in target localization.
- Obtaining diagnostic imaging in the treatment position can optimize image registration.

Treatment Planning

- For both EBRT and brachytherapy, CT-based 3-dimensional planning is favored over 2-dimensional planning to reduce normal tissue dose and better delineate target area.
- Intensity-modulated radiation therapy (IMRT) and image-guided radiation therapy are exploratory and not standard in this setting.
- Dose distribution is calculated with heterogeneity correction and reviewed on all images.

Critical Structures

- Critical structures are site dependent.
  - For extremities, joint spaces and bone are typically in or near treatment volumes. A strip of skin is spared to limit the risk of lymphedema.

- For retroperitoneal sarcomas, the spinal cord, bowel, kidneys, and bladder may be in or near treatment volumes.
- Coverage of the PTV to control disease takes priority; however, limiting dose to normal tissues should be attempted.
  - Less than 50% of a longitudinal strip of skin and subcutaneous tissue to 20 Gy.
  - Avoid full prescription dose to the skin over areas commonly traumatized (elbow, knee, and shin).
  - Less than 50% normal weight-bearing bone to 50 Gy except if involved with tumor.
  - Less than 5% femoral head/neck to 60 Gy.
  - Less than 50% any joint to 50 Gy.
  - Less than 50% anus and vulva to 30 Gy.
  - Less than 50% testis to 3 Gy.
  - V20 lung <37%.

Technical Factors

- For the extremities, 6-MV photons are favored because higher-energy beams may underdose superficial tissues.
- Bolus is applied to surgical scars to increase skin dose.
- Dose homogeneity may be improved with tissue compensators (including physical wedges, dynamic wedges, segmented field technique, and IMRT) and supplementation with higher-energy beams.

EXTREMITY SARCOMA EBRT

Introduction

- Preoperative versus postoperative EBRT are both used, as there are benefits and complications associated with each. Clinical presentations will favor one over the other.

Localization, Immobilization, and Simulation

- When treating an extremity, immobilization of the joints distal and proximal to the target aids in reproducing setup (Figure 11.1a).

Target Volumes and Organs of Interest Definition

- Soft tissue sarcomas (STSs) are generally surrounded by a region of compressed reactive tissue that forms a pseudocapsule, followed by a reactive zone (high T2 signal on magnetic resonance imaging [MRI]) that can harbor microscopic disease.

FIGURE 11.1 Patient with synovial cell sarcoma of the right proximal gastrocnemius. The patient was positioned prone with the left leg "frog-legged" out on a vacuum locking cradle device for CT simulation (a). Using a coregistered MRI for target delineation (b), a 4-field plan with 6-MV photons (c) was used to deliver 50 Gy in 25 fractions (d). Image guidance using kV-cone-beam CT was used for daily localization (e). Wedges were used for the lateral beams, and beams were weighted 3:2, favoring lateral beams.

- Preoperative MRI (T1 with contrast, T2) is necessary for target definition in both the preoperative and postoperative settings.
- Postoperative MRI may be helpful after surgery to identify regions of suspected gross residual tumor.
- Historical block margins modified from O'Sullivan et al. (1), to include use of MRI to define "tissues at risk."
- Preoperative radiotherapy (RT)
    - Gross tumor volume (GTV) = gross tumor defined by MRI T1 plus contrast.
    - Block Margin = GTV + suspicious edema defined by MRI T2 + 5 cm longitudinal margins and 2 cm radial margins
- Preoperative radiotherapy (RT) by Radiation Therapy Oncology Group (RTOG) consensus guidelines for group studies (2).
    - GTV = gross tumor defined by MRI T1 plus contrast.
    - Clinical target volume (CTV) = GTV + 3 cm longitudinal margins (including suspicious edema defined by MRI T2 and shortened beyond the end of the compartment) and 1.5 cm radial margins.
    - Planning target volume (PTV) = CTV + error for setup and organ motion, typically 0.5 to 1 cm.
- Portions of the margins may be reduced if the tumor is confined by an intact fascial barrier, bone, or skin surface.
- Postoperative RT
    - Metallic clips or gold seeds placed during surgery aid in defining the tumor bed.
    - GTV = gross tumor defined by MRI T1 plus contrast.
    - CTV1 = GTV + suspicious edema defined by MRI T2 + 5 cm longitudinal margins and 2 cm radial margins.
    - CTV2 = GTV + 2 cm.
    - PTV = CTV + error for setup and organ motion, typically 0.5 to 1 cm
- Organs of interest include the skin, bone, and joints; testes and ovaries may be considered during treatment planning for proximal thigh lesions.

Treatment Planning

- The minimum dose to a point within the PTV is 97% of the prescription dose, and 95% of the PTV is covered with that prescription dose. No more than 20% of the PTV receives a dose that is 110% or higher than the prescribed dose (Figure 11.1b).
- 3-dimensional conformal RT
    - For distal extremity lesions, opposed lateral fields and multifield arrangements and wedges are used to compensate for changes in extremity thickness (Figure 11.1c).

- More proximal structures often require more complex field arrangements, wedging, or IMRT.
- Planning target volume margins may be reduced with the use of image-guided RT (Figure 11.1d).

Dose/Fractionation

- Preoperative RT
  - 50 Gy/2 Gy/fx to PTV
  - 44 Gy/2 Gy/fx to the PTV if concurrent or interdigitated chemotherapy is used. Interdigitated chemotherapy is typically delivered after 22 Gy (11 fx).
  - Add postoperative boost of 16 Gy for microscopically positive margins and 25 Gy for gross residual disease.
- Postoperative RT
  - 50 Gy in 25 fx to PTV1, followed by a boost to PTV2 to 60 Gy for negative margins, 66 Gy for microscopically positive margins, 75 Gy for gross residual disease.

Intraoperative Boost

- Electron beam therapy may be used in the intraoperative setting to deliver 10 to 12.5 Gy in 1 fx to an area microscopically positive at the time of resection (documented by frozen section).
- Electron energy is typically chosen such that a 1 cm depth or 90% isodose line covers the desired treatment area.

EXTREMITY SARCOMA—BRACHYTHERAPY

Introduction

- Brachytherapy techniques include postoperative low-dose rate or high-dose rate using implanted catheters and other temporary applicators.
- For patients with intermediate to high grade with either positive or negative margins, brachytherapy can be used to boost wide-field EBRT.

Localization, Immobilization, and Simulation

- Metallic clips or gold seeds are recommended to be placed during surgery to aid in defining the residual tumor bed for a positive margin.

Target Volumes and Organs of Interest Definition

- CTV = tumor bed visualized on imaging studies and under direct inspection intraoperatively.
- The American Brachytherapy Society (3) recommends an at least 2 to 5 cm longitudinal margin beyond CTV and 1 to 2 cm spacing between catheters.

Treatment Planning

- HDR brachytherapy catheters are implanted approximately 1 cm apart along the tumor bed, and radio-opaque clips indicate the margins. Optimized treatment planning can be used to deliver a more homogeneous dose.
- In most cases, a single plane implant will be sufficient to cover the CTV.
- Nerve tolerance to high dose per fraction is poor, and HDR should be used with caution when catheters have to be placed in contact with neurovascular structures.
- American Brachytherapy Society guidelines to minimize morbidity with brachytherapy (3).
  - When brachytherapy is used as adjuvant monotherapy, the source loading should start no sooner than 5 to 6 days after wound closure. However, the radioactive sources may be loaded earlier (as soon as 2–3 days after surgery) if doses of less than 20 Gy are given with brachytherapy as a supplement to EBRT.
  - Minimize dose to normal tissues (eg, gonads, breasts, thyroid, and skin) whenever possible, especially in children and patients of childbearing age.
  - Limit the allowable skin dose: the 40-Gy isodose line (LDR) to less than 25 cm and the 25-Gy isodose line to less than 100 cm^2.

Dose/Fractionation

- In general, the dose delivered is related to the dose rate and whether EBRT is used.
- Prescription point is usually 5 to 10 mm from the plane of the implant. If using:
- LDR monotherapy: 45 to 50 Gy/4 to 6 days, 0.35 to 0.6 Gy/h.
- LDR with EBRT: 15 to 25 Gy/2 to 3 days, approximately 0.35 to 0.60 Gy/h.
- HDR fractionated: 3 to 4 Gy daily or twice daily.

Doses of 40 to 50 Gy are given in 12 to 15 fx if the HDR is given alone. If EBRT (45-50 Gy) is added, the brachytherapy dose is limited to 18 to 25 Gy in 4 to 7 fx.

RETROPERITONEAL SARCOMA—EBRT AND BRACHYTHERAPY

Introduction

- Radiotherapy may be given either preoperatively or postoperatively.
- Preoperative RT offers several theoretical and practical advantages over postoperative therapy (Figure 11.2).
  - Optimal knowledge of the extent of disease is possible for treatment planning.
  - Radiotherapy morbidity is usually less.

FIGURE 11.2 Patient with a dedifferentiated liposarcoma of the abdomen. Patient was positioned supine, and IMRT planning using 8 fields of 6-MV photons prescribed to the 98% isodose line was used to deliver 50 Gy preoperative RT; daily IGRT was performed with cone-beam CT.

- Tumor bulk displaces dose-limiting small bowel.
- The bowel is unlikely to be fixed by surgical adhesions seen postoperatively.
- Potentially smaller portal is needed as compared with postoperative RT when trying to cover surgically manipulated tissue.
- There is a possibility for increased complete resection rate secondary to tumor shrinkage.
- Risk of intraperitoneal tumor dissemination may be reduced.
- Intact peritoneal covering provides a physical barrier to early tumor dissemination.
- Displaced normal tissue may permit dose escalation.
- Radiobiologic advantage of intact vascularity and, thus, less tissue hypoxia as in the postoperative setting.
- Disadvantages of preoperative RT include the following:
  - Compromised wound healing after surgery.
  - Delay in surgical resection.
  - Accurate staging may be compromised.

Localization, Immobilization, and Simulation

- Metallic clips or gold seeds are recommended to be placed during surgery to aid in defining the residual tumor bed for a positive margin for intraoperative and postoperative RT.

- Fusion of preoperative imaging is encouraged for postoperative cases
- Saline-filled tissue expander placed at time of resection is safe and may reduce morbidity (4).

Target Volumes and Organs of Interest Definition

- GTV equals the imaging-defined tumor.
- CTV is a 1 to 2 cm margin on GTV.
- PTV expansions are specific to institutional and patient setup parameters.

Treatment Planning

- IMRT may be particularly appropriate, given the range of normal tissues.
- One kidney is commonly within the PTV.
  - Always document the function of the contralateral kidney.
  - Determine the total renal function to ensure adequate residual renal function.
- Normal tissue toxicities of relevance (Table 11.1).

Dose/Fractionation

- Base preoperative/postoperative dose: 45 to 50 Gy/1.8 Gy/fx.
- In the postoperative setting, consider an EBRT beam boost of 5.4 to 9 Gy as deemed safe (Figure 11.3).
- Option as available: intraoperative boost of 10 to 15 Gy using electron-beam therapy or brachytherapy (Figure 11.4).

TABLE 11.1 Retroperitoneal Sarcoma—External Beam Radiotherapy and Brachytherapy: Normal Tissue Toxicities of Relevance

Organ/Fraction of organ	1/3	2/3	3/3	End Point
Stomach	60 Gy	55 Gy	50 Gy	Ulceration/perforation
Kidneys	50 Gy	30 Gy	23 Gy	Nephritis
Liver	90 Gy	47 Gy	31 Gy	Liver failure
Small intestine	50 Gy	–	40 Gy	Obstruction/fistula/perforation
Colon	55 Gy	–	45 Gy	Obstruction/fistula/perforation

FIGURE 11.3 Patient with resected retroperitoneal leiomyosarcoma. Preoperative CT images were coregistered with the simulation CT to aid in target localization (a). IMRT planning using 5 fields of 10-MV photons prescribed to the 98% isodose line was used to deliver 55 Gy to the postoperative CTV (b); daily IGRT was performed with cone-beam CT.

FIGURE 11.4 Patient with leiomyosarcoma of the retroperitoneum. After en bloc tumor resection, the tumor bed received 28 Gy in 4 fx of 7 Gy (>6 hour interfraction interval) prescribed to the 100% isodose line at a depth of 0.5 cm using a Harrison-Anderson-Mick (HAM) applicator. Bowel and abdominal wall were displaced with sterile temporary packing.

HETEROTOPIC OSSIFICATION RT INDICATIONS

- Perioperatively for patients who have undergone orthopedic intervention with a history of prior heterotopic ossification, diffuse idiopathic skeletal hyperostosis, and hypertrophic osteoarthritis, particularly for patients in whom medical treatment with indomethacin is not an option.
- Treat less than 24 hours preoperatively or less than 72 hours postoperatively.

Localization, Immobilization, Simulation

- Positioning: supine with the area to be treated isolated as much as possible (eg, for elbow, may consider arms akimbo).
- Localization: at the site of surgical intervention.
- Immobilization: no formal immobilization techniques are used.
- Simulation: CT simulation, although fluoroscopic simulation is feasible.
- Planning: typically, anteroposterior/posteroanterior fields with dose prescribed to midplane.

Volumes, Dose, and Fractionation

- Volumes (Figure 11.5).
  - Include soft tissue surrounding the joint space.
  - Field size is approximately 7 × 12 cm for the hip.
  - Role of blocking surgical hardware is controversial.
- Dose and fractionation
  - 7 Gy in 1 fx via AP/PA fields with 10 to 18 MV photons.

FIGURE 11.5 Treatment fields from patients with resected heterotopic ossification of the elbow (a) and right hip (b).

REFERENCES

1. O'Sullivan B, Davis AM, Turcotte R, et al. Preoperative versus postoperative radiotherapy in soft-tissue sarcoma of the limbs: a randomised trial. *Lancet.* 2002;359:2235–2241.

2. Wang D, Bosch W, Roberge D, et al. RTOG sarcoma radiation oncologists reach consensus on gross tumor volume and clinical target volume on computed tomographic images for preoperative radiotherapy of primary soft tissue sarcoma of extremity in radiation therapy oncology group studies. *Int J Radiat Oncol Biol Phys.* 2011;81:525–528.

3. Nag S, Shasha D, Janjan N, et al. The American Brachytherapy Society recommendations for brachytherapy of soft tissue sarcomas. *Int J Radiat Oncol Biol Phys.* 2001;49:1033–1043.

4. White JS, Biberdorf D, DiFrancesco LM, et al. Use of tissue expanders and pre-operative external beam radiotherapy in the treatment of retroperitoneal sarcoma. *Ann Surg Oncol.* 2007;14:583–590.

12   Pediatric Radiotherapy

Michael A. Weller and Erin S. Murphy

INTRODUCTION

- There are over 13,000 cases of pediatric malignancies per year.
- The most common include leukemia, central nervous system (CNS) malignancies, and lymphoma.
- Radiotherapy plays an important role in children with solid tumors and, to a lesser extent, childhood leukemia.
- This chapter will focus on photon-based external beam radiation therapy (EBRT). Proton therapy is an option for pediatric malignancies and is currently being investigated at several institutions.

GENERAL PRINCIPLES

- Radiotherapy can affect the development and growth of normal tissues. Because of the young age of children at the time of treatment, understanding normal tissue treatment effects is paramount and techniques should be used to minimize the long-term toxicities.
- Specific dose prescription will be determined by tumor types and treatment approaches, such as preoperative, definitive, or postoperative therapy.

Localization, Immobilization, and Simulation

- Most children younger than 5 years will require daily anesthesia.
  - Techniques include conscious sedation, deep sedation, or general anesthesia.
- Behavioral techniques such as communication via a microphone in the console room or playing a video in the treatment room may facilitate simulation and treatment without anesthesia for cooperative children.
- A pretreatment tour of the simulation and treatment rooms may contribute to a better experience for the patient and family.
- Patient positioning will depend on the treatment site.
- CT simulation $+/-$ intravenous (IV) contrast will enable 3D treatment planning for definition of gross tumor volume (GTV), clinical target volume (CTV), and planning target volume (PTV).
- Immobilization: devices such as thermoplastic mesh for head masks, supine and prone head holders, or vacuum locking (vac-loc) bags allow for easily customizable immobilization.
  - Planning target volume margins should take the degree of immobilization into account.
  - Angled knee sponges and banding of feet aid in reproducing set-up.
    - Special care must be given to working with the anesthesia team for safety of the patient during treatment, with attention to the airway, IV access, and monitors.
- Contiguous spiral CT slices with 3 mm slice acquisition should include the entire treatment volume plus margin and any normal tissue structures that are to be contoured.
- Localization: an isocenter should be placed in the middle of the target volume.
  - Information from operative reports, preoperative and postoperative iodine131-meta-iodobenzylguanidine (MIBG) scintiscan, magnetic resonance imaging (MRI)/CT scans, and positron emission tomography (PET) studies may be incorporated to aid in target localization.

Target Volumes and Organs of Interest Definition

- For help delineating target volumes, one may reference the current Children's Oncology Group (COG) protocols for guidance.
- Structures of interest should be identified and depend on the location of the tumor.
  - Brain: lens, eyes, optic nerves, optic chiasm, pituitary, hypothalamus, brainstem, cochlea, temporal lobes, spinal cord, and cribriform fossa (for whole-brain EBRT).
  - Spine: spinal cord, thyroid, and male or female sex organs.

- Abdomen: kidneys, spinal cord, liver, male or female sex organs, and small bowel.
- Chest: lungs, heart, spinal cord, esophagus, liver, and kidneys.

WILMS TUMOR

RT Indications

- The National Wilms Tumor Studies have developed a multidisciplinary treatment approach that involves upfront surgical staging followed by chemotherapy and radiotherapy when necessary.
- In general, EBRT is not indicated for stage I and II tumors, unless they are unfavorable histologies.
- Regardless of histology, EBRT is indicated for stage III and IV.

Localization, Immobilization, and Simulation

- Positioning: patient should be in supine position with arms above the head or akimbo, especially if lung radiotherapy is necessary.
- Localization: use operative reports and preoperative imaging to delineate operative bed and/or residual disease.
- Immobilization: a device such as a vac-loc bag aids in reproducing set-up.
- Simulation: A 4D or fluoroscopic simulation should be used to determine the extent of motion of the targets and organs at risk, with particular attention to the lungs.

Dose/Fractionation

Special considerations (see Tables 12.1 and 12.2 for summaries)
- Radiotherapy to begin by postoperative day 9.
- Dose per fraction is 1.8 Gy, except when large volumes are receiving EBRT in which case the dose is reduced to 1.5 Gy.
- For patients 16 years or older, 30.6 Gy is prescribed for bone, lymph node, and brain metastases; 19.8 Gy should be delivered to the flank or abdomen.
- Any stage patient with clear cell sarcoma of the kidney should receive 10.8 Gy per the stage III field indications (although stage I is controversial).
- Any stage patient with rhabdoid tumor should receive 19.8 Gy per the stage III field indications. Consider a lower dose for children younger than 1 year.
- For stage V patients, preoperative chemotherapy is usually given. Each tumor should be staged separately. Flank EBRT is recommended for patients with positive margins or positive nodes to a dose of 10.8 Gy. Whole abdominal EBRT is required as per stage III indications (Table 12.1) to a dose

TABLE 12.1 Wilms Tumor: EBRT Indication and Dose/Fractionation

Stage	Histology	EBRT Indicated	EBRT Field	EBRT Dose
I	FH	No		
	UH	Yes	Flank	10.8/1.8 Gy/fx
II	FH	No		
	UH	Yes	Flank	10.8 Gy
III	FH	Yes	Flank: surgical	Flank: 10.8 Gy
	UH	Yes	spillage, flank or peritoneal biopsy, open biopsy WAI (whole abdominal EBRT): cytology + ascites, preoperative tumor rupture, diffuse abdominal surgical spillage, peritoneal seeding	WAI: 10.5 Gy except for diffuse unresectable peritoneal implants: 21 Gy/1.5 Gy/fx
IV	FH/UH	Yes	WLI (whole lung EBRT): lung metastases	12 Gy/1.5 Gy/fx; 10.5 Gy for age <12 y
			Whole brain plus boost: brain metastases	21.6 Gy + boost of 10.8 Gy
			Whole/partial liver: liver metastases	19.8 Gy
			Partial bone: bone metastases	25.2 Gy
			Lymph nodes (unresected)	19.8 Gy
V	FH/UH	Depends on individual tumor stage	Flank: +margins or +LN WAI: as per stage III indications (Consider smaller field for renal sparing as per COG)	10.8 Gy 10.5 Gy

Abbreviations: COG, Children's Oncology Group; FH, favorable histology; UH, unfavorable histology; WAI, whole-abdominal irradiation; WLI, whole-lung irradiation.

of 10.5 Gy. Gross disease should receive a boost of 10.8 Gy. For special considerations of small field renal sparing radiotherapy, see the COG protocols.

- Boost gross residual disease that is greater than 3 cm with an additional 10.8 Gy.
- For diffuse anaplasia, a dose of 19.8 to 20 Gy should be used.
- Irradiating lung metastases is controversial if diagnosed on chest CT, or in the setting of favorable histology or complete response to chemotherapy.
- Persistent focal lung disease 2 weeks after whole lung irradiation (WLI) should be excised or receive a boost of 7.5 Gy in 5 fx.

Target Volumes and Treatment Planning

- If WLI and flank or whole abdominal irradiation (WAI) are required, then the fields can be treated simultaneously or sequentially. If treating simultaneously, the dose per fraction should be reduced to 1.5 Gy. If treating sequentially, typically treat WLI first. In some cases, both the lung and abdomen/flank can be treated with one field. If the areas are treated with two separate fields, the match line should be feathered (moved superiorly or inferiorly 0.5 cm every few fractions) to prevent excess liver and kidney dose (Figure 12.1). See Table 12.2 for typical normal tissue constraints.
- WLI (AP/PA): both lungs are targeted regardless of the location/number of metastases. A 1 cm margin should be added around the entire external pleural surface (Figure 12.2).

FIGURE 12.1 A 4-year-old with bilateral Wilms tumor, stage V, with bilateral pulmonary metastases status post (s/p) chemotherapy and right partial nephrectomy and resection of lymph nodes. Treatment: 10.5 Gy/1.5 Gy/ fx to bilateral lungs and bilateral flank delivered via AP/PA fields using 6-MV photons. Lung and bilateral kidneys are contoured.

FIGURE 12.2 The bilateral lungs received an additional 1.5 Gy in 1 fx, for a total dose of 12 Gy. Right lung contour in blue, left in green.

- Flank (AP/PA): the tumor and involved kidney as determined by the pre-operative CT scan is the GTV. A 1 to 2 cm margin should be added for the CTV; however, if the medial border extends to a vertebral body then the CTV needs to include the entire body plus a margin of 1 cm (Figures 12.3 and 12.4).
- WAI (AP/PA): the superior border is 1 cm above the diaphragm; inferior border is at the bottom of the obturator foramen (with the femoral heads blocked) and the lateral borders are 1 cm beyond the lateral abdominal walls. 3D conformal radiotherapy (3DCRT) or intensity-modulated radiation therapy (IMRT) may be used to boost gross residual disease.
- Whole brain: opposed laterals. For patients who receive a dose of 21.6 Gy and have three or more lesions, a boost of 10.8 Gy may be given by IMRT or single-fraction stereotactic radiosurgery (SRS).

FIGURE 12.3 A 5-year-old with stage I Wilms tumor with diffuse anaplasia, status post (s/p) resection. The flank was treated to 10.8 Gy/1.8 Gy/fx via AP/PA techniques using 6-MV photons prescribed to the 98% IDL. The contralateral kidney is contoured in green.

FIGURE 12.4 Axial CT slice of the plan from Figure 12.3 demonstrating the 100% IDL (yellow) and the 98% IDL (blue). The dose was prescribed to the 98% IDL for optimal coverage of the vertebral body.

■ Liver: for diffuse disease, the entire liver is the target. Otherwise, the lesions as seen on imaging plus a 2 cm margin comprise the target. Of note, if the lesion is solitary and resected with negative margins, radiotherapy is not indicated.

■ Lymph nodes: the metastatic lymph nodes as determined by the pretreatment imaging comprise the GTV. A 2 cm margin is added for the CTV.

■ Bone metastases: the bone lesion as seen on CT or MRI will determine the GTV and a 3 cm margin is added for the CTV.

TABLE 12.2 Wilms Tumor: Normal Tissue Tolerance (per COG protocols)

Structure	Dose Limit, Gy
Small bowel	45
Spinal cord	45
Lung (<50% of the volume is included)	18
Lung (>50% of the volume is included)	15
Kidney (WAI dose >10.5, shield the normal kidney to <14.4 Gy)	19.8
Whole liver	23.4

Abbreviations: COG, Children's Oncology Group; WAI, whole abdominal irradiation.

NEUROBLASTOMA

RT Indications

■ High-risk patients: used to treat primary tumor site and persistent metastatic sites as seen on MIBG scan.

■ Intermediate-risk patients: for recurrent/gross residual disease.

■ Low-risk patients: not indicated after STR or gross total resection.
■ For palliation in stage 4S disease, given to the liver if there is respiratory compromise from rapid hepatomegaly, especially in very young (1- to 2-month-old) patients.

Localization, Immobilization, and Simulation

■ Positioning: the patient should be in supine position with arms above the head or akimbo, especially if lung radiotherapy is necessary.
■ Localization: use operative reports and preoperative imaging to delineate operative bed and/or residual disease.
■ Immobilization: a device such as a vac-loc bag aids in reproducing set-up.
■ Simulation: a 4D or fluoroscopic simulation should be used to determine the extent of motion of the targets and organs at risk, with particular attention to the lungs.

Target Volumes and Dose

■ GTV: the tumor and positive nodal disease as determined by the preoperative CT scan and operative report. A 1 to 2 cm margin should be added for the CTV; however, if the border extends to a vertebral body, then the CTV needs to include the entire body plus a margin of 1 cm (Figure 12.5).
  ■ Dose
    • 21.6 Gy/1.8 Gy/fx daily (COG).
    • 21 Gy/1.5 Gy/fx twice daily (Memorial Sloan-Kettering Cancer Center [MSKCC]).
    • St Jude protocol NB2005 prescribed 23.4 Gy to microscopic and 30.6 Gy to gross disease.
■ Palliative liver: 4.5 Gy/1.5 Gy/fx.
■ Critical structures (Table 12.3).

FIGURE 12.5 A 3-year-old with neuroblastoma, stage IV, status post (s/p) induction chemotherapy and resection (tumor crosses midline, N-myc+, LN+, negative margins after neoadjuvant chemotherapy) and consolidative radiotherapy to the primary disease per COG A3973 protocol. The primary tumor plus a 2 cm margin received 21.6 Gy/1.8 Gy/fx, prescribed to the midplane and delivered with 6-MV photons. COG indicates Children's Oncology Group.

TABLE 12.3 Neuroblastoma: Critical Structures

Organ	Dose Constraint
Liver	≤50% to receive >9 Gy and ≤25% to receive >18 Gy
Contralateral kidney	≤50% to receive >8 Gy and ≤20% to receive >12 Gy
Heart	100% to receive ≤20 Gy and 50% to receive ≤25 Gy
Lung	1/3 to receive ≥15 Gy
Ovaries	Block when possible; consider transposition

Treatment Planning

- Three-dimensional imaging should be used to delineate the target and the normal tissue volumes.
- Beam arrangement: simple AP/PA or 3D planning may be used.

RHABDOMYOSARCOMA

RT Indications

- Indications for radiotherapy are based on IRS grouping (Table 12.4).
- Not indicated for group I embryonal.
- Adjuvant radiotherapy for group I alveolar/undifferentiated and all group II patients.
- Definitive radiotherapy for all group III patients.
- Curative intent radiotherapy to primary and metastatic sites (except bone marrow) for group IV.

Localization, Immobilization, and Simulation

- Positioning: dependent on site of primary
  - For head and neck sites, the patient should be supine with the neck extended.

TABLE 12.4 Rhabdomyosarcoma: IRS Clinical Group Classification

IRS Clinical Group Classification	
Group I	Localized disease, completely resected
Group II	+ microscopic residual or + Regional LN completely resected
Group III	Gross residual after biopsy/resection
Group IV	Distant metastases

Abbreviation: IRS, Intergroup Rhabdomyosarcoma Study.

- For extremities, the patient should be positioned in such a way to enable a beam arrangement that would avoid normal tissues and spare a strip of skin.
- Localization: use operative reports and preoperative imaging to delineate operative bed and/or residual disease.
- Immobilization: a device such as a vac-loc bag aids in reproducible daily set-up. A bite block should be used when treating a head and neck site.
- Simulation: a CT simulation should be performed for 3D planning.

Target Volumes and Dose

- GTV: the tumor and positive nodal disease as determined by the preoperative CT/MRI scan, operative report, and radiopaque clips placed intraoperatively. A 1 to 2 cm margin should be added for the CTV, unless using daily image guidance, which could allow for margin reduction.
- If initial disease responded to chemotherapy and allowed for normal anatomy to resume its natural position, treat initially involved parenchyma but shave CTV off initially uninvolved tissue (eg, lung/bowel) that has returned to normal location and is now in the treatment field.
- Dose (Table 12.5)
- Critical structures (Table 12.6)
- Special considerations
    - Orbit: biopsy alone is sufficient. GTV + 5 mm PTV margin to 45 Gy for group III. Orbital exenteration for salvage only. The patient should be treated with the eye open unless the eyelid is involved.
    - Parameningeal: radiotherapy is given first if there is intracranial extension. The volume is the tumor as seen on MRI + 2 cm margin. Whole brain is used for extensive parenchymal involvement.
    - Vagina and vulva: resection followed by chemotherapy and second-look surgery at week 12 (vulvar) or week 28 (vaginal). Complete vaginectomy

TABLE 12.5 Rhabdomyosarcoma: Dose

Group	Histology	Lymph Nodes	Dose, Gy
I	Poor	–	36 (IRS-V) or 41.4
II	Good	Negative	36 (IRS-V)
	Good	Positive	41.4
	Poor	–	41.4
III	–	–	50.4 (may cone down at 36 or 41.4)
IV	–	–	50. 4 (primary and metastatic sites)

Abbreviation: IRSV, Intergroup Rhabdomyosarcoma Study Group V.

TABLE 12.6 Rhabdomyosarcoma: Critical Structures

Organ	Dose Limit, Gy
Kidney	14.4
Whole liver	23.4
Bilateral lungs	15 (1.5 Gy/fx)
Whole brain ≥3 y old	30.6
<3 y old	23.4
Optic nerve and chiasm	46.8
Spinal cord	45
Gastrointestinal tract (partial)	45
Whole abdomen/pelvis	24 (1.5 Gy/fx)
Whole heart	30.6
Lens	14.4
Lacrimal gland/cornea	41.4

is inappropriate unless there is persistent/recurrent disease. If pathologic complete response (pCR) is noted from biopsy, no further treatment. If biopsy is positive, resect. If unresectable, use radiotherapy either by external beam or brachytherapy.

- Testicular: inguinal orchiectomy and resection of spermatic cord and retroperitoneal lymph node dissection (RPLND) if there are involved nodes on CT or the patient is older than 10 years. RPLND is controversial in the absence of positive lymph nodes (+LN) on imaging studies. Radiotherapy to hemiscrotum, or hemiscrotectomy if the scrotum is violated.

- Bladder: chemoradiotherapy for organ preservation when possible, followed by aggressive surgery for residual or progressive disease.

- Extremity: a 2 cm margin around the mass or tumor bed as defined by MRI. Lymph nodes are treated only when involved. A strip of skin should be spared.

- Thorax: any pulmonary metastases or pleural effusion receive whole lung RT 15 Gy in 1.5 Gy/fx (AP/PA fields); boost residual lung disease (if only a few nodules are present) to 50.4 Gy with 3D-CRT (see Figure 12.2).

- Reproductive organs:
  - For males, consider transposition of contralateral testicle to the thigh before EBRT if scrotal EBRT is required.
  - Consider sperm banking when male is of reproductive age and expected fractionated dose to testes exceeds 2.5 to 3 Gy.

- For females, consider ovarian transposition prior to EBRT. Permanent sterility is age and dose dependent: 12 Gy for prepuberty and 2 Gy for premenopausal.

Treatment Planning

- Three-dimensional imaging should be used to delineate the target and the normal tissue volumes.
- Beam arrangement: depends on the primary site. The use of 3D conformal planning is recommended.
  - Pelvic sites: 4-field box, arcs, AP/PA (spares femoral epiphyseal plates and proximal femurs), or IMRT.

RETINOBLASTOMA

RT Treatment Options

- Radioactive plaques: for solitary 2 to 16 mm basal diameter unilateral lesions located more than 3 mm from the optic disk or fovea, less than 10 mm thick, and for local failure after other therapy.
- EBRT: bilateral tumors, multifocal tumors, tumor location close to the macula or optic nerve, and preserved vision.

Plaque Brachytherapy Technique

- Plaque isotopes include ^{60}Co, ^{125}I, ^{192}Ir, and ^{109}Ru (not FDA approved). The different isotopes provide different isodose distributions and ^{125}I and ^{192}Ir have replaced ^{60}Co.
  - ^{125}I is the preferred isotope in the United States and Canada.
    - ^{125}I physical properties: half-life of 59 days, 28-keV γ-ray energy, and half-value layer of 0.025 mm of lead.
    - Plaques are typically made of gold and range from 10 to 22 mm in diameter.
    - Plaques can be customized according to the tumor shape or location by gluing the ^{125}I seeds to the concave surface of the plaque.
  - Dose: 40 to 45 Gy to the tumor apex, typically delivered over 48 to 96 hours (Figure 12.6); 25 to 30 Gy is recommended after chemotherapy.
- The procedure is performed under general anesthesia.
  - After the conjunctiva is opened, the tumor location is identified by using a transilluminator placed on the globe and then confirmed by indirect ophthalmoscopic globe depression.
  - An inactive plaque is placed with loose sutures in the exact location and is then replaced by the active plaque, which is sutured to the sclera and the conjunctiva is closed.

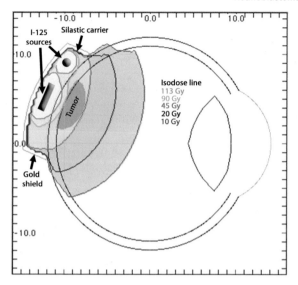

FIGURE 12.6 ^{125}I plaque demonstrating 45 Gy coverage of the tumor outlined in green.

- A lead shield is placed over a patch in front of the eye.
- The patient is brought back to the operating room under general anesthesia for removal of the plaque after the prescribed dose has been delivered.
- RT precautions
  - While the plaque is in place, the patient is kept in the hospital and advised to wear the lead eye shield.
  - The patient's body receives a dose from scattered radiation equivalent to the dose of one chest radiograph.
  - Family members may stay with the patient and are required to wear a radiation badge and ring for monitoring.
  - The patient and room are monitored daily for RT safety.

External Beam RT

Localization, Immobilization, and Simulation

- Positioning: supine with head support.
- Immobilization: a device such as a thermoplast face mask is essential.
- Simulation: a CT simulation should be performed for 3D planning.

Target Volumes and Dose

- CTV: the globe or the entire retina and vitreous with lens sparing
- Dose
  - Typical dose is 45 Gy/1.8 Gy/fx
  - A dose of 36 Gy has been used alone with good local control. Some may consider this dose adjuvantly after chemotherapy or enucleation.
  - Hypofractionation has been used but is generally not recommended because of a higher risk of late effects.

Treatment Planning

- Three-dimensional imaging should be used to delineate the target and the normal tissue volumes.
  - Target should include the entire retina, and 5 to 8 mm of proximal optic nerve.
  - Organs at risk include the contralateral eye and chiasm, pituitary, brainstem, teeth, and upper cervical spine.
  - Planning goals: tumor volume is treated with the 98% line and the orbit is included in the 50% isodose line, with the organs at risk receiving less dose.
- Beam arrangement
  - Historically, orthovoltage was used with a nasal and temporal field used to spare the lens.
  - Three-dimensional and IMRT techniques (using 3–8 beams) are considered superior to the traditional D-shaped field.
  - Stereotactic radiosurgery and proton therapy are also being investigated.

PRIMITIVE NEUROECTODERMAL TUMORS

RT indications

- This family of tumors is also known as embryonal tumors or primitive neuroectodermal tumors (PNETs), and the most common include medulloblastoma, supratentorial PNETs, and atypical teratoid rhabdoid tumors.
- Treatment for these tumors typically includes maximal surgical resection followed by chemotherapy and craniospinal EBRT.

Localization, Immobilization, and Simulation

- Positioning: prone or supine position.
  - Extend the neck to avoid divergence of the spinal field into the oral cavity. The head should be supported by a rest and positioned relative to the body to minimize cervical spine curvature and skin folds.

- Arms at the sides with the shoulders lowered to allow junction shifting.
- Prone
  - Advantages: allows direct visual confirmation of field junctions and good alignment of the spine.
  - Disadvantages: uncomfortable, technically difficult to reproduce, and does not allow for easy intubation with anesthesia.
- Supine
  - Advantages: comfortable, easier to reproduce, allows for intubation.
  - Disadvantages: inability to visualize bony landmarks for visual setup confirmation (eg, visual verification of skin gap for field match)
- Immobilization: custom mold or vac-lock bag should be used for reproducible setup, with the goal of a straight spine. Thermoplast head mask should be used to immobilize the head.
- Localization: the patient is scanned (3 to 5 mm slices) from the vertex to the midfemurs. The isocenter is placed in the brain field, and triangulation points are marked on the mask. The patient is also marked at the upper thorax and pelvis for alignment.
- Simulation: computed tomography simulation is recommended to obtain 3D volumetric information of target and critical normal tissues.

Treatment Planning

- Two-dimensional field arrangement: planning begins with simulation of the spinal field first.
  - Spine: PA field from C4-7 interspace to 1 cm beyond the thecal sac (visualized on sagittal MRI), extending laterally to cover transverse spinal processes
    - Controversy regarding the caudal end of the field: some question if it needs to be widened by up to 1.8 cm to encompass the increasing distance between nerve root exits as they move inferiorly down the spine, making coverage of the sacroilliac joints unnecessary.
  - The lowest cervical interspace possible is used for the superior edge of the field to accommodate subsequent "feathering" of the junction.
  - If unable to encompass the entire span with a single field, 2 fields may be used with a junction gap calculated with the following equation to match fields at a specified depth and avoid convergence of beams too superficially (Figure 12.7a):

$$\text{Separation} = \frac{1}{2}\left(\frac{L\,1\times\text{Depth}}{\text{SSD1}}\right) + \frac{1}{2}\left(\frac{L\,2\times\text{Depth}}{\text{SSD2}}\right)$$

Separation = gap length at skin surface
L = length of the PA spinal field

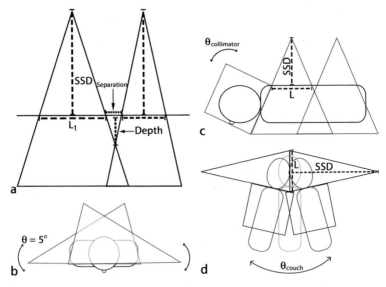

FIGURE 12.7 Depiction of cranial spinal setup. (a) Similar triangles used for gap calculation. (b) Gantry rotation used to avoid divergence through the contralateral lens. (c) Lateral view demonstrating collimator rotation to match the divergence of the superior spine field. (d) Superior view demonstrating the table kick used to avoid the divergence of the whole-brain field into the spinal field.

> Depth = depth at which the field edges superimpose
> SSD = source-surface distance of the PA spinal field

- Whole-brain field: German Helmet technique (see Chapter 13, WBRT) with 5° posterior tilt to spare the contralateral lens (Figure 12.7b). Blocks are designed to ensure adequate coverage of the cribriform plate and middle cranial fossa (typically 1 cm margin). If using fluoroscopic simulation, an arrow is used to mark the right bony canthus and a marker on left bony canthus.
- The collimator is rotated to match the divergence of the superior border of the spine field with the inferior border of cranial fields (Figure 12.7c).

$$\theta_{collimator} = tan^{-1}\left(\frac{1}{2} \times \frac{L}{SSD}\right)$$

$\theta_{collimator}$ = angle of collimator rotation
L = length of the PA spinal field
SSD = source-surface distance of the PA spinal field

- Divergence between the brain and spinal field is accounted for by rotating the couch toward the gantry to match the superior border of the spine field with the inferior border of cranial fields along the R-L axis (Figure 12.7d).

$$\theta_{couch} = tan^{-1}\left(\frac{1}{2} \times \frac{L}{SAD}\right)$$

θ_{couch} = angle of couch kick
L = length of the lateral cranial fields
SAD = source axis distance of the lateral cranial fields

- Field matches: with the use of collimator rotation and an independent jaw technique, the cranial and spinal fields may be directly abutted (light fields). Many radiation oncologists prefer a gap between the cranial and spinal light fields; thus, a gap of 0.5 cm is allowed on most protocols. The match line should be moved superiorly by 0.5 to 1 cm after each 8 to 9 Gy (usually done once per week). Also, a penumbra broadening "match line wedge" or a dynamic wedge may be used to minimize inhomogeneity.

- 3D field arrangement: conformal treatment planning with CT simulation if available is preferred for beams-eye-view. Field arrangement and target coverage is similar to 2-dimensional planning, but calculations are not required, as collimation and table rotations are determined with the treatment-planning software. Intensity-modulated radiation therapy treatment planning offers dosimetric advantages over traditional 3D-CRT in both dose homogeneity and normal tissue sparing.

Target Volumes and Dose

- GTV: gross residual tumor and/or the walls of the resection cavity at the primary site from the initial and postoperative/preoperative RT imaging.

- CTV: GTV with an added margin to cover subclinical microscopic disease that is anatomically confined (ie, the CTV is limited to the confines of the bony calvarium and tentorium). There are several CTVs to take into account.

  - CTV whole brain: extends anteriorly to include the entire frontal lobe and cribriform plate. Inferiorly, the CTV1 should be at least 0.5 cm below the base of the skull at the foramen magnum.

  - CTV spine: entire cord and thecal sac. To extend laterally to cover the recesses of the entire vertebral bodies, with at least a 1 cm margin on either side. The superior border will be the junction with the whole-brain field. The inferior border will be 2 cm below the termination of the subdural space.

- CTV posterior fossa boost: inferiorly from C1 vertebral canal through the foramen magnum, laterally to the bony walls of the occiput and temporal bones and superiorly to the tentorium cerebelli.
- PTV: in order to account for the daily setup error, the additional margin defining the PTV may range from 0.3 to 1.0 cm.
- Dose prescription
  - Average-risk medulloblastoma: CSI to 23.4 Gy/1.8 Gy/fx followed by posterior fossa boost to 54 Gy/1.8 Gy/fx.
  - High-risk medulloblastoma and supratentorial PNET: CSI to 36 Gy/1.8 Gy/fx followed by posterior fossa boost of 18 Gy/1.8 Gy/fx to 54 Gy.
- Organs at risk (Table 12.7).

TABLE 12.7 Primitive Neuroectodermal Tumors: Organs at Risk

Structure	Dose Limit/Special Considerations
Supratentorial brain (left and right)	Avoid hot spots.
Cochlea (left and right)	32 Gy/(better visualized on CT bone window)
Hypothalamus	45 Gy/(better visualized on MRI if available)
Pituitary	45 Gy
Eyes (left and right)	50 Gy
Lens (left and right)	7 Gy
Optic nerves (left and right)	50 Gy (may go up to 59.4 Gy if necessary)
Optic chiasm	50 Gy (may go up to 59.4 Gy if necessary)
Spinal cord	50 Gy (No more than 50% of the cervical spinal cord between C1 and C2 should receive more than 54 Gy).
Cribriform plate	Better visualization and decreased error in localization with CT simulation. Important to ensure it is included in the whole brain field.
Ovaries	Be aware of dose to this structure and consider transposition or half beam blocking the inferior spinal field.
Thyroid	Try to avoid matching through this structure.

Abbreviation: CT, computed tomography.

▪ Secondary image sets: fusion of preoperative and postoperative MRI image sets to planning CT scan should be performed. These complimentary imaging modalities assist in delineating target and critical structures as detailed above.

CRANIOPHARYNGIOMA

Radiotherapy Indications

▪ Radiotherapy is not indicated after gross total resection.
▪ Adjuvant radiotherapy is indicated after subtotal resection.
▪ Immediate postoperative radiotherapy provides better outcomes than does EBRT at time of recurrence.
▪ Radioactive colloid may be used for primary or recurrent large cystic tumors.

Localization, Immobilization, and Simulation

▪ Positioning: the patient should be in supine position with arms at the sides or across the chest.
▪ Localization: use operative reports and preoperative and postoperative MRI to delineate operative bed and/or residual disease.
▪ Immobilization: aquaplast face mask.
▪ Simulation: a CT simulation should be performed for 3D planning.

Target Volumes and Dose

▪ GTV: postoperative residual disease and deflated cyst as identified on MRI.
▪ CTV: GTV + 1 to 2 cm margin.
▪ Other investigative approaches have included a CTV = GTV + 5 mm and PTV = CTV +3 mm when using imaging guidance with weekly MRI. Imaging during treatment is recommended, as the cysts may grow beyond the field during treatment.
▪ Dose
  ▪ 54 to 55.8 Gy/1.8 Gy/fx.
  ▪ 11 to 12 Gy in 1 fx prescribed to the 50% IDL may be considered for SRS.
  ▪ Intracavitary radionuclide dose is 200 Gy to cyst wall with ^{32}P or ^{90}Y (β emitters)
▪ Critical structures (Table 12.8)

TABLE 12.8 Craniopharyngioma: Critical structures

Organ	Dose Constraint (Whole or Partial Organ), Gy
Retina	45
Lens	10
Optic nerve	50
Optic chiasm	50
Brainstem	1/3, 60; 2/3, 53; 3/3, 50
Pituitary	45
Temporal lobes	1/3, 60; 2/3, 503; 3/3, 45

Treatment Planning

- Three-dimensional imaging should be used to delineate the target and the normal tissue volumes.
- Single-fraction stereotactic radiosurgery can be considered in the postoperative or recurrent setting when the tumor is 5 or more mm away from the optic chiasm.

13   Palliative Radiotherapy

Gaurav Marwaha, Andrew D. Vassil,
and Gregory M. M. Videtic

GENERAL PRINCIPLES

- Palliative radiotherapy balances symptom control while minimizing therapy-related adverse effects.
- Patient's performance status, physical limitations, natural disease history, and previous therapies should all be considered when designing an appropriate radiation course.
- Custom immobilization techniques, hypofractionation, brachytherapy, intensity-modulated radiation therapy (IMRT), intracranial stereotactic radiosurgery (SRS), stereotactic body radiotherapy (SBRT), and radiopharmaceuticals may be considered when individualizing therapy.

Localization, Immobilization, and Simulation

- Positioning: assessing a patient during consultation can facilitate identifying the most comfortable and reproducible position for simulation that achieves acceptable beam arrangements (Figure 13.1a and b). Soft materials

FIGURE 13.1 Patient with pain caused by right axilla metastases from melanoma. Simulation with patient supine, on soft sheep's wool table cover, arms akimbo (a). Anteroposterior (AP) port showing the painful area delineated with radio-opaque wire taped to the patient's skin (b).

on the tabletop, such as lamb's wool, may be used to improve patient comfort.

◼ Immobilization: minimally restrictive devices, such as tape and straps, and more rigid devices, such as thermoplastic mesh or vacuum-locking bags, allow for easily customizable immobilization.
  ◼ Planning target volume (PTV) margins should take the degree of immobilization into account.
  ◼ Angled knee sponges and banding of feet aid in reproducing setup.
  ◼ SBRT requires a high degree of immobilization, typically using items such as thermoplastic molds, vacuum-locking bags, infrared localization, and intrafraction orthogonal radiograph position confirmation.
  ◼ Medication: pretreatment with analgesic and antiemetics can improve comfort during simulations and treatment.
  ◼ Localization: radiopaque markers may aid in correlating pain with simulation images (Figure 13.1 a and b).
    • Fluoroscopic or computed tomography (CT) simulation is typically used.
    • Information from operative reports, magnetic resonance imaging (MRI) and positron emission tomography (PET) studies may be incorporated to aid in target localization.

- Isocenter: for photon simulation isocenter is placed at least D_{max} depth from the surface and typically in a central or deeper location. For electron simulation, the isocenter is placed at the skin surface.

Target Volumes and Organs of Interest Definition

- Target volumes and normal structures: International Commission on Radiation Units & Measurements (ICRU) guidelines should inform target delineation but may not be as strictly applied, as mandated by the patient's specific clinical needs.

Treatment Planning

- Dose prescription: a depth or location (eg, isocenter or midplane) for dose prescription allows for rapid, simple treatment planning.
- 3D conformal radiotherapy (3DCRT): when clinically necessary to reduce high doses to non-target tissues. Oblique field angles may help avoid spinal cord and other sensitive tissues.
- IMRT: may be favored in the setting of retreatment, for nontarget tissue sparing in selected cases, but usually comes at the expense of longer treatment times.
- Multifield and arc-beam SBRT: high conformality with dose escalation may be favored in the setting of retreatment or specific clinical scenarios.
- Electron fields: electrons are well suited to treatment of superficial lesions.
  - Choice of electron energy relates to field size and desired prescription isodose line.
  - Templates for electron cone inserts may be generated during the examination of a patient or through the use of simulation images.
  - Custom electron cone inserts may then be made and port films acquired as part of the simulation process.
- Critical structures: regions for dose limitation depend on target location.
- Beam energies: depends on target geometry and relation to surrounding structures.
- Heterogeneity correction: not conventionally used
- Field matching: gantry and table rotation and using a half-beam block can help match fields for patients undergoing a radiation course near a previously treated field or in anticipation of matching fields in the future.

BONE METASTASES

Indications

- Techniques used to treat pain or disability from bone metastases typically use standard photon or electron external beam radiotherapy.

- Prophylactic irradiation of metastases may prevent fractures in high-risk areas, typically at the acetabulum and/or proximal femur.
- Hemibody radiation therapy and radiopharmaceuticals may be considered for widespread symptomatic disease.

Localization, Immobilization, and Simulation

- Positioning: comfort, reproducibility, and ease of setup favored
  - Supine positioning is used for most situations.
  - Arms often at the sides but raised above the head typically when treating thoracic metastases.
  - Angled devices that elevate the chest may be used for patients with respiratory difficulties.
- Localization: delineating painful areas with radiopaque markers taped to the skin can help ensure that clinically involved regions are encompassed by the radiation field.
- Immobilization: for treatments of extremities, immobilization of the joint distal to the region of interest (with a vacuum-locking bag) aids in reproducing setup.
- Gantry and table rotation may be used to minimize divergence, particularly for rib lesions to avoid unnecessary lung radiation.

Target Volumes and Organs of Interest Definition

- Lesions correlating with painful areas delineated at the time of simulation are encompassed in the treatment volume.
- Radiolucency seen with lytic lesions; radiopacity is seen with blastic lesions, and areas of fracture are targeted. Regions of FDG PET avidity and marrow infiltration/cortical destruction seen on MRI may also be included.
- Pelvic metastases are often treated in a manner that will allow field matching if additional treatment is needed. This is accomplished by using landmarks such as the sacroiliac joint, pubic symphysis, and greater trochanter to be used as points of reference if future treatment is necessary (Figure 13.2).
- For spine metastases, target volumes typically include one vertebral body above and below areas felt to be causing symptoms.
- After medullary fixation, the whole surgical field, all hardware, and methylmethacrylate stabilizing the bone are considered at risk for recurrence and are encompassed in the radiation field.

FIGURE 13.2 Patient with pain caused by a left femoral head/neck metastasis from prostate cancer. This patient previously received 70 Gy prostate bed salvage radiotherapy. AP portal targeting femoral head/neck.

Treatment Planning

- Field arrangements: Varies depending on the region to be treated and the physical limitations of the patient and matching positioning. Examples of typical field arrangements include the following:
  - AP/PA (extremities, sacrum, and pelvis)
  - PA (lumbar, thoracic spine)
  - En face electron (skull, scapula, sternum, rib, and clavicle)
  - Lateral and oblique parallel opposed (cervical spine and rib)
  - Wedged pairs (rib and superficial lesions)

Dose/Fractionation

- The patient's performance status, natural history of the patient's disease, previous therapies, and inherent sensitivity of a given histology should all be considered when determining a radiation dose and fractionation.
  - A dose of 8 Gy delivered in a single fx with 6- to 10-MV photons or electrons is effective in most situations. A dose of 20 to 30 Gy delivered in 5 to 10 fx may also be considered.
  - A dose of 30 Gy delivered in 10 fx is safe and typically given 10 to 14 days after surgical procedures such as spinal decompression and medullary fixation.
- Reirradiation: treating beyond normal tissue tolerance should be avoided, unless mandated by the patient's need. Consider alternative radiotherapy techniques.

- Hemibody radiation: This technique is useful for patients with widespread painful bone metastases.
    - Fields are divided at the umbilicus or L4/L5 with an extended SSD with 6- to 10-MV photons.
    - Transmission lung blocks limit midline lung dose to 6 to 7 Gy.
    - 6 Gy delivered to the upper body and 8 Gy delivered to the lower body in 1 fx.
    - Alternatively, 15 Gy in 5 fx, 20 to 30 Gy in 8 to 10 fx given 3 fx per week.
    - The other half of the body is treated 6 to 8 weeks later.
- Radiopharmaceuticals
    - May be considered for patients with multiple blastic lesions from breast and prostate cancer.

Radiopharmaceutical	T1/2	Dosage (IV)	Notable
Strontium-89	50.5d	4 mCi or 0.04-0.06mCi/kg	Beta-emitter; incorporates into bone hydroxyapatite (like calcium) for 100d; works best in blastic mets
Samarium-153	1.9d	1 mCi/kg	Beta-emitter; don't give if renal insufficiency
Radium-223 (Alpharadin)	11.4d	50 kBq/kg	Alpha-emitter; FDA approved for metastatic hormone-refractory CaP only

Abbreviations: CaP, prostate cancer; FDA, Food and Drug Administration; IV, intravenous.

SPINAL CORD COMPRESSION

Indications for Radiation

- Nonsurgical patients, postoperative patients (generally within 14 days of surgery or adequate healing time).
- To improve pain, local control, ambulatory ability.

Localization, Immobilization, and Simulation

- Supine or prone (driven by patient comfort).
- Localization: delineating areas of cord compression with MRI and/or CT spine with radiopaque markers.
- Immobilization: see General Principles.

Volumes and Treatment Planning

- Fields
  - Lateral: cover width of vertebral body with 1 to 2 cm margin, including areas of paravertebral tumor extensions.
  - Superior/inferior: 1 (if using MRI) or 2 cm (if using CT) vertebral body above and below epidural metastasis.
- Beams
  - Energy based on patient anatomy, 6 MV most commonly utilized.
  - Opposed laterals for cervical lesions (avoid esophagus).
  - PA only for thoracic $+/-$ lumbar lesions.
  - AP/PA for lumbar lesions approaching midline.
  - Prescribe to depth of 5 to 10 cm, based on patient's anatomy (Figure 13.3).
- Dose/Fractionation
  - 20 Gy/5 fx, 30 Gy in 10 fx are commonly used schedules.
  - 8 Gy x1 for patients with short life expectancy or with poor performance status.
  - Alternative fractionation schemes include: 16 Gy/2 fx (one week split), 37.5 Gy/15 fx, 40 Gy/20 fx.
  - All schemes show equivalent survival and functional outcomes. Long course (30 in 10 or higher) may improve local control and progression free survival.

SBRT FOR SPINE METASTASES

Introduction

- Typically used for patients with high performance status, low volume of disease, and radiobiologically resistant disease, with symptomatic disease recurrence in a previous radiation field.
- Potential advantages of SBRT: bone marrow preservation by treating limited volumes, convenience of fewer patient visits compared with fractionated therapy, less interference with ongoing chemotherapy treatments, use as a decompressive therapy for those with epidural compression, and noninvasive alternative to surgery.
- Disadvantages of SBRT: cost, complexity, patient tolerability, delay in time to initiation of treatment, field size limitations, duration of radiation delivery, necessary specialized equipment, and benefits over conventional radiotherapy remain to be demonstrated.
- The following is based in part on the Radiation Therapy Oncology Group (RTOG) 0631 protocol.

Localization, Immobilization, and Simulation

- Positioning: due to the prolonged duration of treatment fractions, a comfortable supine position must be found.
- Localization: systems that relate patient position to the table and isocenter are used.
  - A frame with a stereotactic localization coordinate system may be used.
  - Depending on the method of image guidance to be used at the time of treatment, fiducial markers (eg, infrared reflective) may be placed on the frame and patient.
- Immobilization: rigid immobilization systems are used because of the necessary setup precision.
  - Custom devices providing multiple points of contact are used.
  - Examples include a vacuum-locking bag or thermoplastic mask for cervical spine treatments.
- Thin-slice simulation CT (typically 2 mm) is coregistered with high-resolution magnetic resonance images (T1 with gadolinium contrast and T2 sequences) to aid in target delineation.
- Image-guided radiotherapy (IGRT): internal landmarks (eg, bone and fiducial implants) verifying positioning should be less than 2 mm from the simulation position. IGRT devices to verify patient position may involve orthogonal imaging, cone beam computed tomography (CBCT), electronic portal imaging devices, and CT-on-rails systems.

Target Volumes and Organs of Interest Definition

- Definition of the PTV
  - Involved vertebral body, pedicles, and gross disease including paraspinal masses (Figure 13.3).
  - Transverse processes, lamina, and spinus process are included when the disease is located in posterior vertebral elements.
  - A space of 3 mm or greater between the spinal cord and PTV should be present.
  - Paraspinal mass should be 5 cm or less.
- Critical structures
  - Spinal cord: delineated on MRI; 5 to 6 mm superior and inferior to the level of the CTV, depending on CT slice thickness.
  - Normal organs should also be delineated when these structures are in the beam path.

FIGURE 13.3 Patient with vertebral body metastases previously irradiated with conventional technique. PTV (blue line) and spinal cord (yellow line) delineated on axial and sagittal planes; 15 Gy (purple) and 10 Gy (green) isodose "clouds". Nonopposed, coplanar beams with 6-MV photons used.

Treatment Planning

- Photon energy: typically, 6-MV photons are used, given the decreased penumbra and reduced exit dose relative to higher energy photons.
- Dose rate: to limit treatment time, 800 monitor units/minute or higher is desired.
- Beam arrangement: multiple posterior nonopposed coplanar beams or posterior arc beam fields with the beam isocenter at the center of the PTV. Noncoplanar beams and IMRT may be used for irregularly shaped targets.
- Prescription point: prescription is typically to the 80% to 90% isodose line (IDL). A dose greater than 105% of the prescription dose should not be outside of the PTV.
- Normal tissue limits: 10% of the spinal cord (5–6 mm above and below the PTV) should be limited to receive 10 Gy. Less than 0.35 cc of the spinal cord should receive 10 Gy. Reconstructions with isodose displayed should be reviewed to ensure that no region is receiving a higher than acceptable dose, particularly the spinal cord. Refer to the RTOG 0631 protocol for dose restriction guidelines.

Dose/Fractionation

- For de novo treatments, 16 Gy is prescribed to include at least 90% of the PTV.
- When treating a volume within a previously irradiated field, 14 Gy is used.

BRAIN METASTASES—WHOLE BRAIN RADIATION THERAPY (WBRT)

Introduction

- WBRT is used as a single modality or in conjunction with surgery, SRS, and chemotherapy.
- A slightly larger field ("German helmet") is also used, especially when there is a concern for leptomeningeal spread of disease or with posterior fossa lesions.

Localization, Immobilization, and Simulation

- Positioning: the patient is positioned supine with the head in a neutral position. Radiopaque markers are placed at the fleshy canthus bilaterally.
- Localization: head rotation is corrected before making the immobilization mask by viewing the position of the laser lines on structures such as the nose and auditory canal. Fluoroscopy or scout image may be taken to confirm head position.
- Immobilization: a thermoplastic mask is made.
- Lateral radiographs or CT images are acquired.

Target Volumes and Organs of Interest Definition

- Definition of the PTV
  - Clinical setup of the field is done to include the entire brain; if CT planning is used, review of axial images can help ensure that the entire brain is included and dose to nontarget structures is minimized.
  - Attention is paid to ensure adequate margin on the cribriform plate and temporal lobes.
  - The posterior half of the orbits are included in a German helmet field, in an effort to include all meningeal surface (Figure 13.4b and d).
  - Critical structures
- Normal tissues such as the lenses, posterior oropharynx, and posterior neck soft tissues may be avoided by blocking with primary collimator rotation, 5-HVL (half value layer) cerrobend blocks, or multileaf collimators.

Treatment Planning

- Photon energy: typically, 6-MV photons are used.
- Beam arrangement: opposed lateral fields, with the isocenter placed at midplane; for German helmet plans, a 5 degree gantry rotation is used to create anteriorly nondivergent fields that avoid treating the lenses (Figure 13.4b and d).

FIGURE 13.4 Right lateral standard WBRT field (a) and German helmet field (b). Isodose distribution displaying the 100% (yellow), 107% (red), and 95% (blue) isodose lines for WBRT (c) and German helmet fields (d).

- Fields
  - Standard WBRT fields: the collimator is rotated to block the anterior orbit and tissues anterior to the skull base; a 1 cm border anterior to the skull base is typically adequate to ensure coverage of the temporal lobe (Figure 13.4a).
  - German helmet field: a 5 degree posterior gantry rotation minimizes divergence into the lens. The collimator is kept at 90 degrees, the C2-3 interspace is used for the inferior boarder (Figure 13.4b).
  - The field is opened to provide margin superiorly and posteriorly at least 1 cm beyond the skull (ie, "flash").
  - Blocking at the C1-2 interspace may be used for whole-brain fields for the purpose of potentially matching fields in the future.

■ Hippocampal Sparing (investigational only)
  ■ May decrease neurocognitive side effects of WBRT (ie, learning, memory, spatial processing).
  ■ IMRT is required for delivery. See recently completed RTOG 0933 protocol for contouring guidelines.

Dose/Fractionation

■ No fractionation schedule is superior to another based on randomized studies, and RT prescription often reflects patient performance and institutional practice.
■ In the United States, 30 Gy/3 Gy/fx is commonly used and is also used after surgical resection of metastases.
■ Typically, 37.5 Gy/2.5 Gy/fx is used for patients who will or have received SRS (1).
■ 20 Gy/5 Gy/fx: often for patients with poor performance status and active extracranial disease.
■ 20 Gy/2 Gy/fx: in the setting of repeat WBRT after a patient has previously received 25 to 37.5 Gy.
■ Appropriateness criteria have been produced by the American College of Radiology (2).

BRAIN METASTASES—STEREOTACTIC RADIOSURGERY (SRS)

Introduction

■ SRS uses multiple beam paths to provide high doses of radiation with rapid dose fall-off for intracranial metastatic lesions typically 40 mm or less in maximum dimension.
■ SRS requires extremely precise immobilization, imaging, and radiation delivery.
  ■ Delivery systems: Gamma Knife® (GK, Elekta, Stockholm, Sweden) radiosurgery system; CyberKnife® (Accuray, Sunnyvale, CA); modified traditional linear accelerator (eg, Novalis, Palo Alto, CA).

Localization, Immobilization, and Simulation

■ Immobilization: frame-based and "frameless" techniques are used
  ■ A rigid metal frame is attached to the skull with four screws. The frame provides immobilization; stereotactic localization systems attach to the frame.
  ■ Attention is paid to the location of the targets in reference to the frame position, to avoid placing the frame directly over the target lesion(s).

■ Frameless immobilization uses a thermoplastic mask, infrared fiducial markers, and orthogonal radiograph guidance during radiation delivery.

■ Localization: high-resolution CT and MRI studies (1 mm slice thickness) are conducted with the patient supine and the frame locked to the imaging table.

　■ Image sets are coregistered using the stereotactic fiducial coordinate system attached to the frame (Figure 13.5a).

　■ A skull scaling device is used to make external head contour measurements for GK planning to assess beam path length in tissue. This is particularly useful when the entire head is not imaged, and surface data are not available.

　■ Other treatment planning systems may use the head contour delineated from simulation CT.

■ Immobilization: the frame attaches to the treatment table, immobilizing the patient's head.

Target Volumes and Organs of Interest Definition

■ Definition of the PTV

　■ Metastatic lesions are delineated on MRI coregistered to simulation CT.

　■ Target volumes should be at least 5 mm away from the optic chiasm and nerves.

■ Critical structures

　■ The optic chiasm is delineated on MRI coregistered to CT; coronal views aid in identifying the optic chiasm.

FIGURE 13.5 Stereotactic coordinate system used for image registration (a); typical isodose distribution in a GK plan encompassing metastatic lesion with the 50% IDL (b).

Treatment Planning

- GK and CyberKnife systems use spherical points of radiation dose ("shots" for GK, "nodes" for CyberKnife) generated by fixed circular collimators.
  - The "shots" or "nodes" can be abutted with forward planning to generate irregularly shaped isodose distributions.
- The GK Perfexion® system uses multiple focused "sectors" of varying collimator sizes to generate irregularly shaped isodose distributions.
- CyberKnife systems use fixed circular collimators and deliver "nodes" from multiple gantry positions with the use of a linear accelerator mounted on a robotic arm. A "step-and-shoot" technique is used; that is, radiation is not delivered while the robotic arm is moving.
- Linear accelerator-based treatment typically uses 6 to 8 arced photon fields. Varying the fixed circular collimator ("cone") size or multileaf collimator (MLC) shape ("dynamic arc"), number and position of isocenters, number of arcs, arc angle, degree of arc rotation, and weight of each arc can help shape the isodose distribution to conform to the target. To improve dose conformity to the target, IMRT may be used.
- After planning is complete, dose-volume histogram (DVH) and isodose distributions on all images should be reviewed to ensure that areas of unacceptably high dose do not fall on critical normal structures, such as the optic chiasm.
- Dose is prescribed in a manner such that the 50% IDL encompasses that target lesion for GK systems (Figure 13.5b); the 80% isodose line is used for linear accelerator-based systems. This is the "median marginal dose," that is, the median dose at the target margin.
- Conformity index is the prescribed isodose volume divided by the target volume and should be have a value between 1 and 2.
- Homogeneity index is the maximum dose divided by the prescribed dose and should be a value less than 2.

Dose/Fractionation

- Per RTOG 90-05, a single fx of 24 Gy for lesions 2 cm or less, 18 Gy for 2.1 to 3.0 cm, and 15 Gy for 3.1 to 4.0 cm are used.

MALIGNANT OBSTRUCTIONS AND BLEEDING

Introduction

- Debilitating and life-threatening events can be caused by intrinsic and extrinsic airway obstruction, superior vena cava (SVC) compression, and esophageal compression and bleeding.
- EBRT can provide durable symptom relief and may be combined with other therapies.

- Brachytherapy may also provide durable relief but should not be combined with concurrent chemotherapy.

Localization, Immobilization, and Simulation

- Positioning: in most situations, patients are simulated supine with arms above the head.
    - In cases of severe airway and superior vena cava (SVC) obstruction, patients may be more comfortable on an angled board to elevate the thorax.
    - An upright, seated position can be used for patients who cannot tolerate a supine position.
- Localization: oral contrast (such as gastrografin) helps identify esophageal obstruction and may identify tracheoesophageal fistula.
    - Tracheoesophageal fistula is not a contraindication for EBRT; however, brachytherapy is believed to be unsafe in this setting.
    - Endoscopic placement of a 6 to 10 mm diameter catheter is done for brachytherapy procedures. Distance and active length measurements are made at the time of catheter placement and verified at time of simulation. Surgical clips may be placed endoscopically to delineate the extent of disease in cases of esophageal obstruction.
- Immobilization: rigid immobilization is typically not needed. For patients in a seated position, a rigid back rest is used for consistent setup. For brachytherapy, the catheter is marked at the level of the incisors and taped to the patient's face to keep it from migrating.
- CT simulation is preferred over fluoroscopic simulation to better visualize the extent of disease.

Target Volumes and Organs of Interest Definition

- Definition of the PTV
    - Gross disease (GTV) causing obstruction should be included with a 1.5 to 2 cm combined CTV/PTV expansion.
- Critical structures
    - Normal organs should also be delineated when these structures are in the beam path.

Treatment Planning

- EBRT: typically, 6-MV fields are used with anteroposterior/PA fields for most sites.
- Brachytherapy: 3D planning is preferred (Figure 13.6).
    - Active length for brachytherapy is determined by the length of disease seen at endoscopy and on simulation CT.

FIGURE 13.6 Patient with bleeding from an esophageal cancer now being treated with brachytherapy. Isodose distribution for prescription normalized to a depth of 0.5 cm. Brachytherapy source dwell positions are noted with red dots.

■ Source dwell time optimization may be used to expand coverage at the distal portions of the active length.
■ Active length should be 10 cm or less.

Dose/Fractionation

■ For esophageal brachytherapy, 10 to 14 Gy high dose rate (HDR) in 2 fx 1 week apart is prescribed at a 1 cm radius from the midsource position. Also, low dose rate (LDR) may be used to deliver 20 to 25 Gy in a single fx at 0.4 to 1 Gy/h (3).
■ For endobronchial brachytherapy, 15 Gy HDR prescribed in a similar fractionation and depth as esophageal brachytherapy may be used.
■ EBRT dosing for situations of bleeding, bronchial and SVC obstruction: include hypofractionated regiments such as 17 Gy/8.5 Gy/fx separated by 1 week or 20 to 30 Gy/3 to 4 Gy/fx.
■ EBRT dosing for esophageal obstruction is 30 Gy/3 Gy/fx; more protracted radiation courses and/or combined chemotherapy reflect patient status and clinical judgment.

SKIN AND SOFT TISSUE METASTASES

Introduction

■ Techniques for treating soft tissue metastasis include photon or electron fields and may involve SBRT
■ Hyperthermia may serve as an adjunctive therapy in situations of reirradiation of superficial soft tissues such as a chest wall recurrence.
■ Radioactive yttrium-90 microspheres may be considered for treatment of liver metastases.

Localization, Immobilization, and Simulation

- Head and neck skin and nodal metastasis: position the patient supine with head extended and shoulders down; a thermoplastic mask is made and the patient is imaged from vertex to carina or inferior extent of disease (eg, mediastinal disease). Bolus may be applied under the mask; thus, the mask will aid in keeping bolus material in place during treatment.
- Pancoast syndromes: position the patient supine, head rotated contralateral to the disease, arms above the head or at side; image from mastoid tip to inferior aspect of thorax (to ensure imaging of entire lung tissue).
- Pulmonary and mediastinal metastasis: position the patient supine with arms above the head or at the side; image from midneck to inferior aspect of thorax (to ensure imaging of entire lung tissue). In cases of oligometastatic pulmonary disease, SBRT may be considered.
- Liver metastases: position the patient supine with arms above the head; image from thoracic inlet to iliac crests; 4D-CT may be considered in an effort to reduce PTV margins, particularly for patients who have received prior radiation therapy near the target region. For oligometastatic disease, SBRT may be considered.
- Pelvic malignancies: the patient is positioned supine with arms across the chest; image from the level of the L1 vertebral body to the lesser trochanter.
- Skin metastases: bolus material, typically 1 cm thick, may be custom cut to encompass volumes delineated by radiopaque marker with additional 2 to 3 cm margin. Simulation imaging may be conducted with bolus over the region to be treated; alternatively, bolus material may be designed using the treatment planning software, then custom cut.
- CT simulation is generally preferred.

Target Volumes and Organs of Interest Definition

- Definition of the PTV
  - Gross disease (GTV) identified on CT simulation causing obstruction and palpable disease should be included with a 1.5 to 2 cm combined CTV/PTV expansion.
  - Skin, head, and neck: areas clinically involved as identified by patient history, physical examination, and imaging is delineated at the time of simulation. Regional lymphatics may be included in the treatment field depending on histology and factors such as performance status and prior radiation fields.
- Critical structures
  - Normal structures surrounding the PTV (eg, parotid glands, spinal cord, esophagus, normal lung tissue, kidneys, and liver) should be delineated and considered in treatment planning.

Treatment Planning

- Generally, 3D planning with 6- to 10-MV photons or electrons of energy to encompass PTV within the 80% to 100% IDL is used.
- Electron templates may be designed without simulation imaging for well-defined, palpable, superficial lesions that have recently been characterized by volumetric staging studies, such as CT. Target areas may be marked on the patient's skin with ink, a transparent film is overlaid, and the area is traced. An electron cone insert is made from the traced area and appropriate electron energy is chosen based on desired target dimensions.

Dose/Fractionation

- In most situations, for patients with skin or soft tissue metastases, 20 to 30 Gy/3 to 4 Gy/fx can be used.
- Alternatives include:
  - Melanoma and renal cell carcinoma: 5 Gy/fx, twice weekly to a total dose of 30 Gy.
  - Liver metastases (whole or partial liver): 10 Gy delivered in 2 fx separated by 6 to 24 hours (4).
  - Adrenal metastases: 30 Gy/2.5 to 3 Gy/fx.
  - Splenomegally from leukemia: 5 to 10 Gy delivered in 1-Gy fx given 3 times a week.
  - Pelvic malignancies: 10 Gy in 1 fx, may be repeated after 4 weeks.
  - Skin metastases: 8 Gy in 1 fx.

REFERENCES

1. Andrews DW, Scott CB, Sperduto PW, et al. Whole brain radiation therapy with or without stereotactic radiosurgery boost for patients with one to three brain metastases: phase III results of the RTOG 9508 randomized trial. *Lancet.* 2004;363:1665–1672.

2. Videtic GM, Gaspar LE, Aref AM, et al. American College of Radiology appropriateness criteria on multiple brain metastases. *Int J Radiat Oncol Biol Phys.* 2009;75:961–965.

3. Gaspar LE, Nag S, Herskovic A, et al. American Brachytherapy Society (ABS) consensus guidelines for brachytherapy of esophageal cancer. Clinical Research Committee, American Brachytherapy Society, Philadelphia, PA. *Int J Radiat Oncol Biol Phys.* 1997;38:127–132.

4. Bydder S, Spry NA, Christie DR, et al. A prospective trial of short-fractionation radiotherapy for the palliation of liver metastases. *Australas Radiol.* 2003;47:284–288.

Index